MEDITATION FOR BEGINNERS

8 Weeks To A New Life

-The African Edition

By

DEMETRIUS IRICK

PROVOKE
PRESS

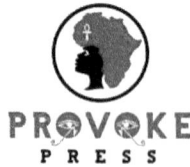

Copyright ©2020 by Demetrius Irick

by sales or promotional materials. The advice and strategies contained herein may not be suitable for every situation.

This work is sold with the understanding that the publisher and author is not engaged in rendering medical, legal, or other professional advice or services. If professional assistance is required, the service of a competent professional person should be sought. Neither the Publisher nor the author shall be liable for damages arising here.

The fact that an individual, organization, or website is referred to in this work as a citation and or potential source of further information does not mean the author or the publisher endorses the information the individual organization or website may provide or recommend they or it may make. Further, readers should be aware that Internet Websites listed in this work might have changed or disappeared between when this work was written and when it is read.

Provoke Press
ISBN: 978-0-9857903-8-7

In Praise of Meditation for Beginners, 8 –Weeks to a New Life

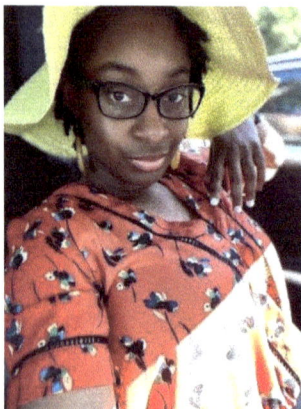

"I was new to meditation and not sure how to get into it or even if I had time for it. Everything was at my own pace and easy as I went forward. Everything was detailed and steps broken down for anyone to follow. It's full of information that made me excited for each week to come."

-Danielle Wilson

"Finished the book and it was absolutely amazing! We love the feel of it as a knowledgeable & teaching tool for meditation. What we loved most was your transparency in how meditation has transformed your life."

-Darrick and Leslie Goodman, CKYT

"This book is just what we need for our Awakening and the information is an amazing asset in navigating your conscious journey. Choose to be invested in your growth and healing by using this great guide as a starting point for creating your routine to develop a better you. Thank you Demetrius for listening to your guides and being in alignment with your Devine Assignment. May Ntr continue to bless you and clear your path as you align mind, body and soul to receive what is truly yours! Ase

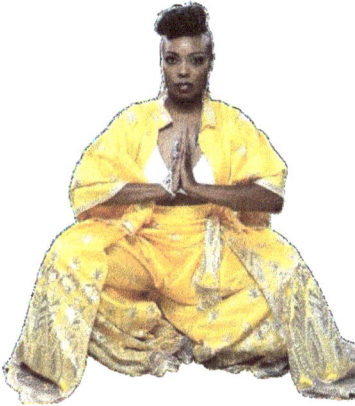

-Tamara Shanell, Holistic Practitoner

Acknowledgments

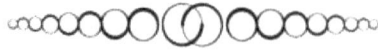

Love begins, or should begin, at home and for me that is Thomas and Sara Irick. I can comfortably say without them I would still be seeking love instead of writing about how it's been crucial in my development of self-love. That also means Karen, if all wives loved as you do there would be fewer men looking to fill their voids in another. Lastly, that's Daijah & Jaclyn who are now exploring new worlds out of the nest but I know they are safe and grounded ready to tackle whatever the world may present to them. I am truly blessed, grateful and appreciative for all the experiences life has bestowed upon my life.

I am indebted to the host of professionals who I've gleaned much knowledge and wisdom, which has shaped my life. Among them are Cheikh Diop, John Jackson, Nathan McCall, Anthony Browder, Runoko Rashidi, Malcolm X, Muata Ashby, Iyanla Vanzant and Yirser Ra Hotep to name a few.

This book is dedicated to all of individuals that know they need to invest in their selves but don't know where to start. Meditation is the gateway to a life of fulfillment and reaching beyond your wildest dreams.

"In the beginner's mind there are many possibilities; in the experts mind there are few."

-Shunryu Suzuki

Zen Mind

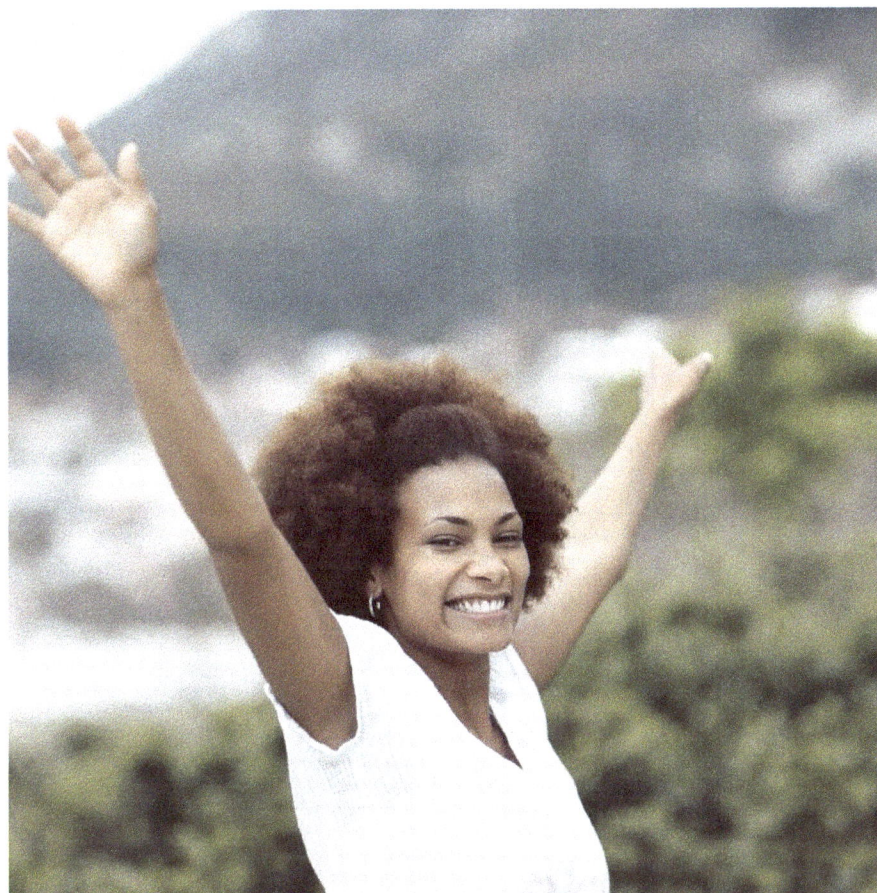

"The only way to get what you really want is to let go of what you don't want."

-   Iyanla Vanzant

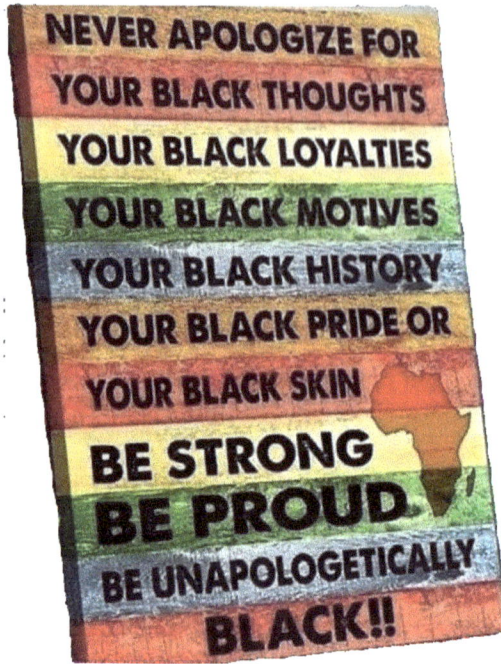

NEVER APOLOGIZE FOR
YOUR BLACK THOUGHTS
YOUR BLACK LOYALTIES
YOUR BLACK MOTIVES
YOUR BLACK HISTORY
YOUR BLACK PRIDE OR
YOUR BLACK SKIN
BE STRONG
BE PROUD
BE UNAPOLOGETICALLY
BLACK!!

"It's easier to raise healthy children, then to rebuild a

broken man"

-Fredrick Douglas

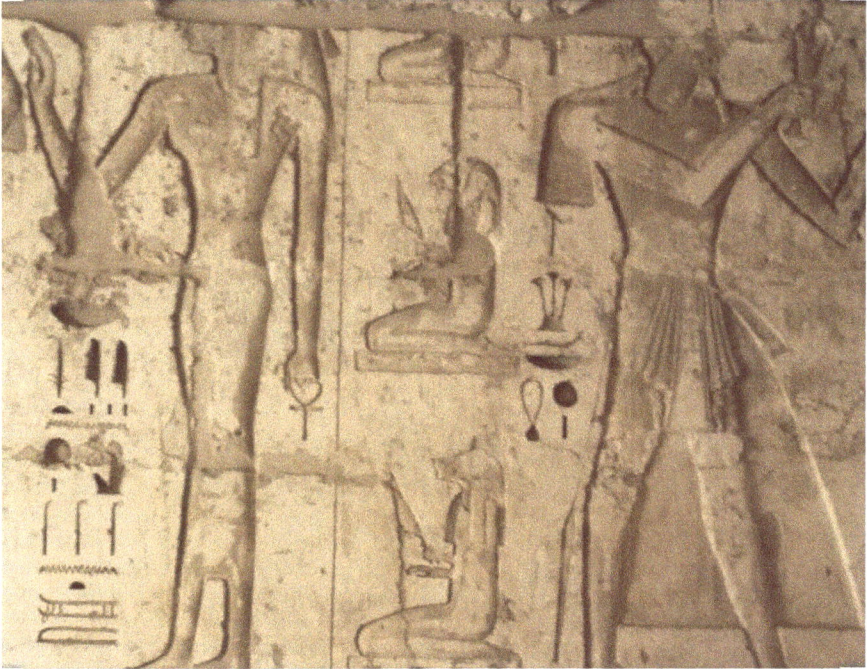

" In any situation you have the right, power and ability to choose your experience."

-Iyanla Vanzant

Contents

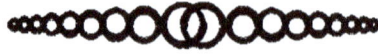

Testimonials

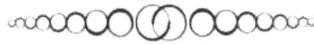

"Meditation is internal freedom. It is a necessary fuel that is free to all if we understand how to use it. It protects us in the physical and it transcends with us spiritually. It is activated by the breath, the Life Force. Meditation constantly transforms us, our union with one another, and how we deal with life as a whole. It provides clear skies when the world is overcast."

> -   Leslie Goodman, CKYT

"Meditation has taught me to have patience within myself. Sitting in a comfortable position and breathing was never easy for me. What I didn't initially understand is the importance of having consistency in sitting still and breathing for a preset amount of time was helpful. There were many times my thoughts were not calm, painful even. I found taking things one-step at a time was key. Acknowledge the act of sitting, the time and the breath first…the calming of the mind comes with consistency."

> -   Darrick Goodman, CKYT

Demetrius Irick

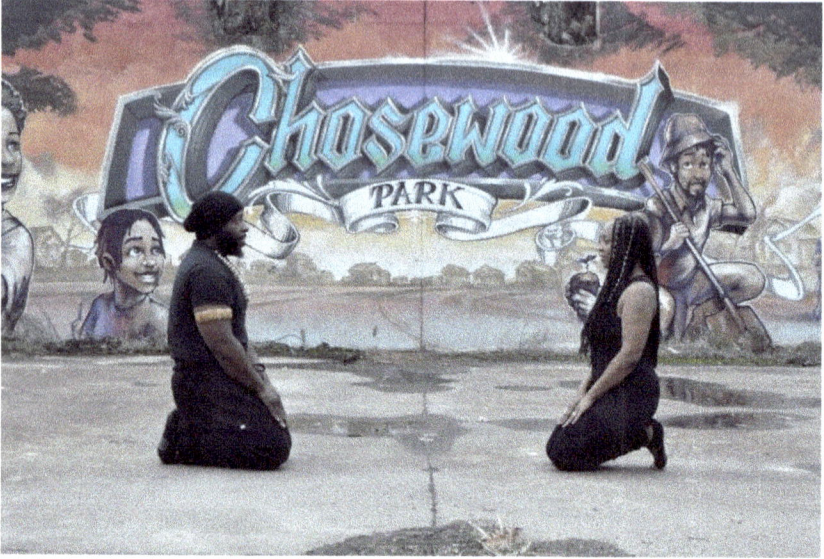

[SESH 3 POSE] (A Kemetic YogaTM Meditation Pose)

Darrick Goodman and Leslie Goodman are Certified Kemetic Yoga™☐ Teachers at the 200HR level as well as founders & owners of Black Silt Yoga ®☐ LLC. Practicing and teaching Kemetic Yoga ™☐ together as husband and wife, they are soul mates sharing divine union. Darrick and Leslie currently teach Kemetic Yoga™☐ online and in person with specialized teaching to Couples, Community, and Corporations. For information on classes and events please contact us using the detailed information below.

Contact Info
☐: (833)BLK-SILT/ (833)255-7458
: blacksiltyoga.com
✉@: darrickandleslie@blacksiltyoga.com
Social Media
IG: @blacksiltyoga FB: Black Silt Yoga LLC Black Silt Yoga ®☐ LLC
Darrick Goodman, CKYT Leslie Goodman, CKYT

"Meditation is a major key to life. It wasn't until I started incorporating my connection to breathe in my spiritual practice that I unlocked my true connection to spirit and my higher consciousness. It is because of me using different modalities of meditation I was able to find exactly what was needed for different parts of my life. In the beginning it may seem challenging and even frustrating to disconnect from your oh so busy mind but trust beloved with time, consistency and patience you will master this ancient tool that will unlock so many doors in your minds."

–Tamara Shanell, Holistic Practitioner
The Healing Chamber
www.thehealingchamber.org
IG: @thehealingchamber

Demetrius Irick

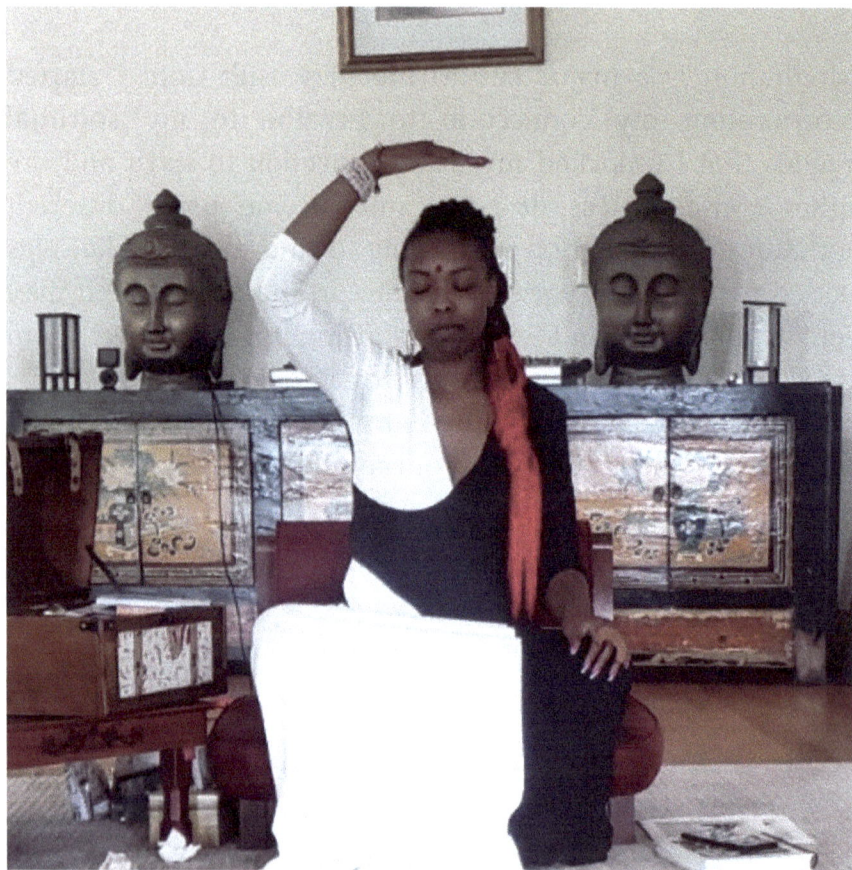

Over the past 5 years, yoga and meditation have developed into my favorite way to access peace of mind. I grew up with a mother who struggled with mental health challenges and a father who was very practical and not so much emotionally expressive. I began seeing myself struggling in the same capacity without knowledge of how to heal or the emotional awareness to express my current state at the time. My emotions were moving more and more out of balance, as the polar effects of anxiety and depression started consuming my life. Yoga started as a means of maintaining flexibility, but now yoga and meditation are my means of maintaining balance in every single aspect. Some of our life experiences can be chaotic, overwhelming, saddening and destructive. Strengthening my practice allows me to have useful tools to navigate the intense energy we may face with the options to root myself in a grounding meditation so I'm not moved in the storm, to utilize specific poses for tapping into the power centers we have within or to travel through a yoga flow when I need to create movement in areas of my life. My practice is healing, sacred and a way to draw closer to the Source. Cultivating my practice is honestly one of the greatest gifts and opportunities I've experienced thus far.

-Rachel E. the Goddess, Yoga Instructor, Labor Doula, Registered Nurse

Demetrius Irick

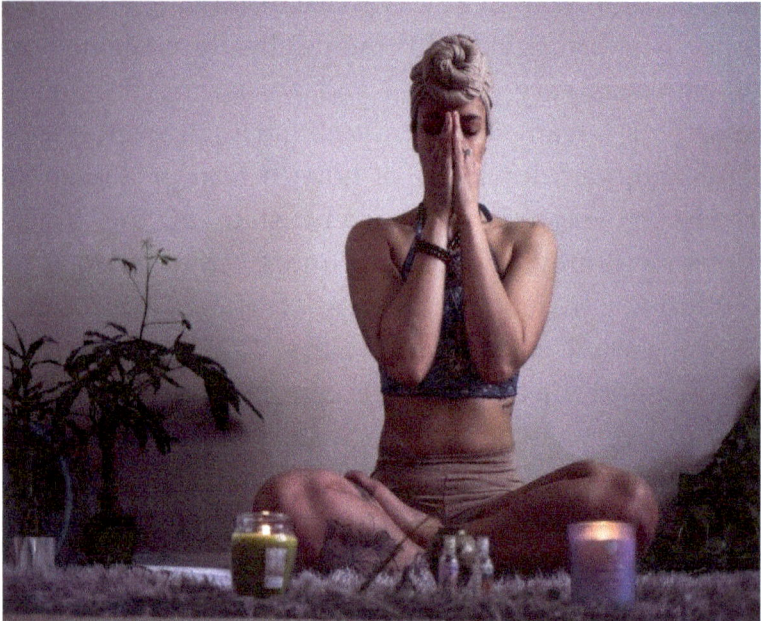

Contact Information:
Instagram - @rachel.e.thegoddess/ @ahyokaheals
Website - www.ahyokaheals.org

Introduction

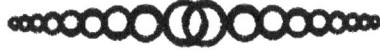

This book was created with one goal in mind and that's to change your life using the art of meditation. Meditation has been around for thousands of years and the benefits are documented in countless scientific sources. The health benefits include lowering blood pressure, better concentration, slowing down dementia, reduced stress & anxiety, depression and the list go on & on. Although, meditation does have some religious affiliation it's not solely a religious thing. Meditation will not conflict with your religious belief but it will enhance anyone's spiritual practice.

I began practicing meditation after the death of my grandmother in 1994. At the time I was nineteen and wasn't aware of what meditating was, but I was led to the stillness that gave me inner peace during a time when I was emotionally unstable. I remember meditating outside in the midst of the sun and feeling so at home, a feeling I never felt while in church. I was seen as an outcast for embracing this art, called names, bullied and badgered in the process. I eventually succumbed and stopped practicing all together.

Fast-forward twenty 23 years another life event shattered my normal coping process. The divorce of an 18-year marriage and dealing with the emotional rollercoaster left me with few options in dealing with my triggers. It was then I begun the tedious process of self-care and mental health restoration. It was then that I found my abandoned practice once again. I started simply by taking a few short but deep breaths and that calmed my anxiety down. I had a panic attack while at work that led me to seek counseling. I found speaking to a neutral individual resulted in the clarity I needed to invest in my mental health. Historically, the subject of mental health is frowned upon in my community, but this was a true blessing and thus the birthing of this book.

It was through the art of meditation that I slowly began the process of mental peace of mind and wanted to encourage everyone to take advantage of the free tool of meditating.

It's my wish for you that this book becomes your motivation to begin a simple practice of self-acceptance and self-love. If the mere idea of meditating feels uncomfortable or scary it's okay soon you will find it to be your slice of heaven. Exploring the unknown territory of anything new is usually different, awkward, and stressful only because it' different. Think of anything that you've done that was new or difficult at first and now you can do it with your eyes closed. I thought about riding a bicycle as a child, the nervousness of driving a car the first time or getting your driver's license, asking someone out on a date, or just going on your first date. Contrary to stereotypes you won't turn into a hippie, have to change your friends, or pack up and have to move to reap the benefits of your meditation practice. This is a gift to give to yourself and nobody even needs to know you are meditating, but you just might love it so much that you will want to teach your friends and family.

There needn't be any big mystery or drama about the process itself, and there's no right or wrong way of doing it. There are simply different techniques that can be used as tools to help you focus and quiet your mind, and we'll work with some of these as the weeks unfold. This will allow you to choose which method works best for you as an individual. We have all seen the vision of the yogi sitting crossed legged wearing robes and perhaps meditating in a cave. This is not what meditation is about for most of us and starting with an unrealistic idea of what meditation is about won't make it an enjoyable experience for you. I still have a hard time quieting my mind and I find that my meditation practice is more fulfilling for me while I'm in nature or near water personally. Again, what I intend on doing with this book is to help you develop a meditation practice that's right for you. Don't worry by the end of the book it will be something you feel comfortable doing.

Practice Meditation Already?

For those of you who already have a meditation routine, we've come to depend on the way our practice enhances our lives. We've discovered an ever-present source of inner peace and wisdom from which we can now draw strength, courage, clarity, and compassion. It has become easier to respond to situations from a calm and grounded place, rather than acting out old dysfunctional patterns. We're also better able to navigate our lives in alignment with our own needs and goals. By giving ourselves space to simply be ourselves, many of the distractions from other people's agendas melt away. For many of us, meditation has become an important way to take really good care of ourselves. You wouldn't dream about leaving your house in the morning without bathing or brushing your teeth and this is eventually how you will feel about your practice. Meditation will give you the confidence and the strength you will need each day and a sense of accomplishment to get the day started.

So, let's begin…8 weeks to a better, healthier you!

What is Meditation?

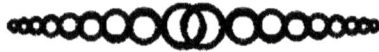

Meditation is a practice where an individual uses techniques such as mindfulness, breathing techniques, object focus, and countless other techniques to train the individual's attention and awareness to give a calm and stable state of being. Meditation is an ancient art that increases calmness, physical relaxation, improves psychological balance, and enhances overall health and mental well-being. The connection of the mind and body through this practice focuses on the interactions with the brain, mind, body, and their innate behaviors.

Meditation is all about the journey and not the destination. There will be days where you will not be able to focus your mind and it will wander about but it's okay. It's a practice you have to do it! Meditation is one of the unique arts as it's both a skill and experience. Let's talk a little about what meditation is not... it's not about "emptying the mind", or "stopping one's thoughts." Our mind's sole purpose is to think therefore trying to make it stop is not part of the process. We mediate to be the observer of those thoughts, to understand them more clearly. Meditation is not about becoming a different person or a new person. Although, the practice does make you more comfortable with yourself building your self-esteem and worth which will have a positive effect on your demeanor and outlook. It's this inner-work that will yield you becoming the best version of yourself. Meditation does not guarantee relaxation, serenity, or bliss but all can be a by-product of good meditative practice.

Demetrius Irick

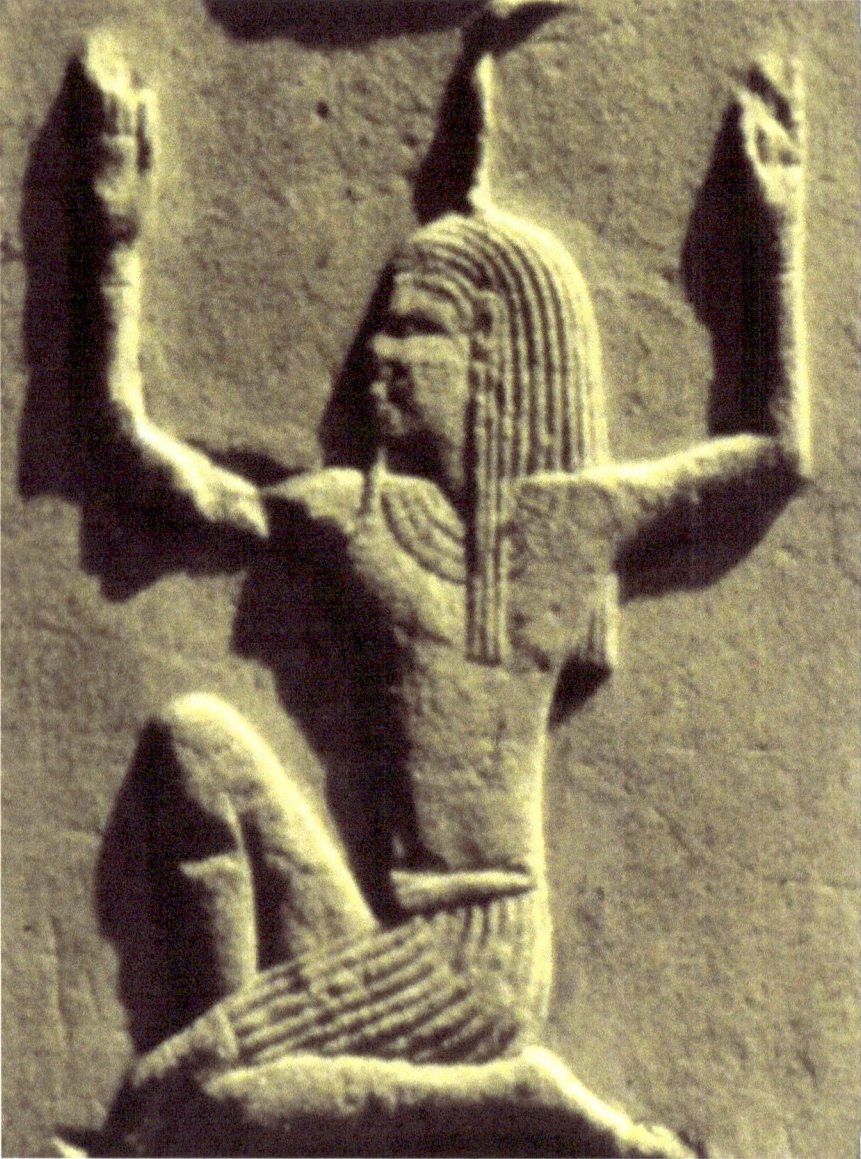

"Look inside to the shadows of your life for the biggest

breakthrough"

-Demetrius Irick

History of Meditation

The art of meditation was practiced in Ancient Kemet the land of the blacks over 5,000 years ago, which predates any worship associated with the Indian or Buddhist traditions of Yoga. It's a Yoga discipline that was practiced to reach spiritual enlightenment. Enlightenment is a term used to describe the highest level of spiritual awakening. Our Ancestors understood the human mind and its complex nature. They understood the strengths and weaknesses individuals would face when they aren't in Maat or balance.

Our Ancestors understood that the art of purifying the mind, and physical disciplined is needed to discover our enlightenment. Peace, contentment, and joy are only achieved when one reaches their sense of purpose or discover there meaning for life. The Ancient Africans created the first civilization, taught leaders from around the world and

Demetrius Irick

spearheaded advancements in science, astrology, medicine, and meditation & yoga is no different.

Health & Meditation

Research studies indicate that meditation combined with deep breathing exercises treats many mind and body disorders. There are many benefits to starting a meditation practice, but a few are things like substance abuse, anxiety, depression, muscle spasms, anger, high blood pressure, and heart disease to name a few. The fact that when the practitioner engages in meditation, there is a level of calmness that brings relaxation to the body and also increases the psychological balance in each individual that practices are worth giving it a try.

Research has linked a regular practice of mediation to reduced stress, improvement of the immune system's function, and increase gray matter in the brain.[1] It's this increase in the gray matter that contributes to increased attention, focus and concentration found in the ACC (anterior cingulate cortex) which is deep inside the forehead behind the frontal lobe. It's the ACC area that minimizes our desire to react to situations and gives us the strength to respond instead of reacting. Imagine being able to decide how you are going to respond to any of the emotional triggers that set you off in the past. Imagine having a choice on how you want to react to the feelings of hurt, despair, disappointment, regret, verbal abuse, etc. Meditation puts the control back in your hands on how you decide to entertain every situation. Studies have shown that the nervous system begins responding differently to stressful situations and our brain and body go into a healing mode as oppose to survival mode. The metabolism drops, stress level goes down and the brain is fully developed and functioning at higher levels of functionality. During, your practice you will find that a higher level of alpha waves are present, which enables more concentration and productivity which is great for getting things done. Want to write a book? Be a better leader, develop better parenting skills, learn to cook, check off things on your bucket list by starting a meditation practice, and gain momentum towards your new way of living.

Spirituality & Meditation

Meditation is the connection to the Creator, Source, or Higher Power. It gives the practitioner a sense of awareness that they are already united with the ONE SOURCE. It's through meditation that the countless number of connections we share with the "ONE" becomes crystal clear. Through this silence and observation, we become more in tune with all of life that surrounds us…from the smallest (ant) to the largest (whale).

Because of the distractions in our society and life we rarely take the opportunity to sit still long enough to bask in all the connections we share with the creation and each other. Most of the popular religions confine the Creator to a "Being" or "a something" that is separated from us. This tool makes us aware that God, The Supreme, or whatever name you choose to assign it exists in the fiber of our bones, through our breath and every atom of our life. It reminds us that the "ONE" is reflected in nature and every living creature. I believe that meditation is a confirmation that God is omnipresent, which in a nutshell means the Creator of human existence is everywhere, and in everything living thing. Therefore, meditation is merely the time in thought that connects you to that Source…so tap into your connection with Source today.

"A lot of people fear being in the dark. They fear the unexpected that the blanket of darkness provides. Meditation forces you to sit in that darkness in your mind and soul and provides clarity for the unexpected thoughts that arise from your soul. Fear of what is inside of you…is what keeps you from the commitment to better yourself."

-Demetrius Irick

Beginner Meditation

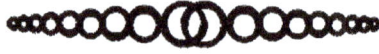

Week 1

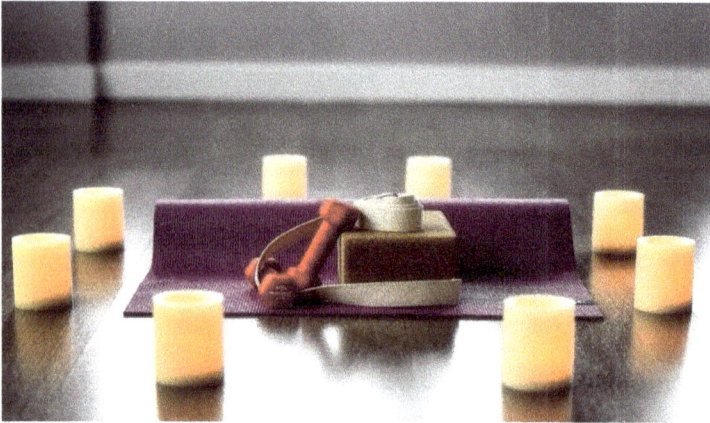

Now, with that being said let's get rid of some stereotypical thoughts of meditation. Meditation is a journey that is well worth the time you invest in it. The secret is finding something that works for your lifestyle. You want to establish a routine that will enable you to commit regularly. No one has the keys to what will work for you…only YOU! This book will

give you different techniques for you to unlock the process
that works best for you.

Getting Started

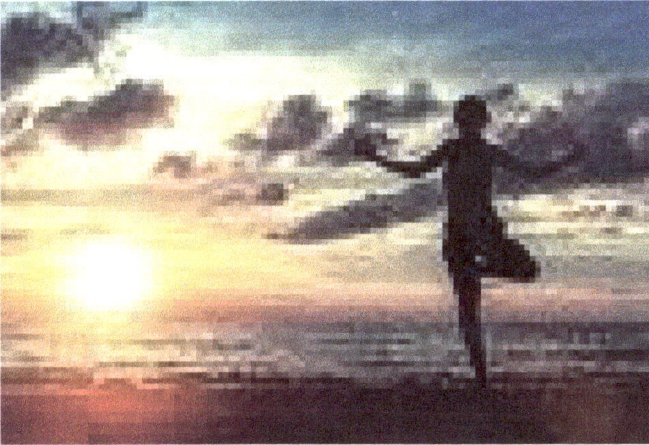

Regular consistent practice will yield the best results as stated
earlier. Just like anything new you will get better with time
and practice. Try not to be hard on yourself as you begin this
process. You're the only one who can take this journey and
the best place to start is right where you are. At first, you may
not be able to sit for more than a few minutes and that's ok,
but soon you'll be meditating for 5, 10, 20, or 30 minutes with
ease. The idea is to get a habit started, so aim for consistency

(i.e., meditating 5-10 minutes a day, every day) over longer sessions (i.e., meditating for a whole half hour, every once in a while).

You generally don't need to purchase anything to start a meditation routine and no special equipment or clothing is required as long as you're comfortable. Some people buy what's known as a meditation cushion to get proper support and elevate the pelvis placing the hips above the knees just to hold the spine in the proper position but it's certainly not necessary. Some also find that lighting a candle or incense signals an official start to their meditation and this can help the mind to focus. (Chimes, singing bowls and bells may also be used for this purpose.)

Next week, we'll be exploring some particular meditation practices that use candles and incense, so if you don't already have these around your home, you may want to get some that you'll enjoy working with.

It is not uncommon for inspiring ideas and solutions to emerge during meditation. I always have a journal with me so

I can write down the wonderful ideas that come to mind during my sessions. You may want to experiment with this as well. It can help your mind return to silence.

How should I sit when I meditate?

Let's explore a few different ways of sitting. You may be familiar with the classic lotus position or half-lotus position (see photos below) in which many long-term meditators are pictured. This position is ideal because it allows for a balanced and unobstructed flow of energy throughout the energy centers of your body. Some people cannot sit this way because they are physically inflexible or having back or knee issues. You may find that over time you gain the flexibility to meditate in the lotus position; or, you may simply decide that an alternate posture works better for you. Please don't feel that you have to sit in these positions right away, it can take time to build up to it.

Demetrius Irick

The key to remember when selecting your meditation position is that you'll want to keep your back straight and your palms open or facing upward.

There are a few different positions for your hands to take during meditation, but for now, keep your hands open toward the sky and have them rest on your thighs, knees, or ankles depending on what is comfortable once you are in position with the rest of your body.

 Whether you decide to lay down, sit against a wall with your back aligned, or just sitting in a chair…we need for you to be comfortable to minimize any distractions that come from physical exertion from being in discomfort.

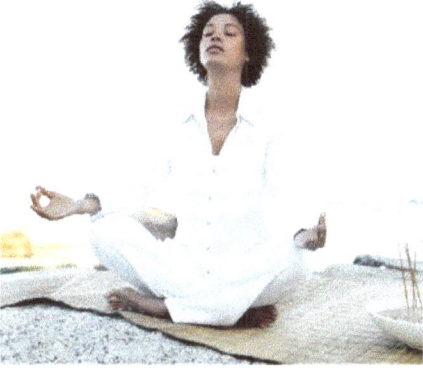

Half Lotus

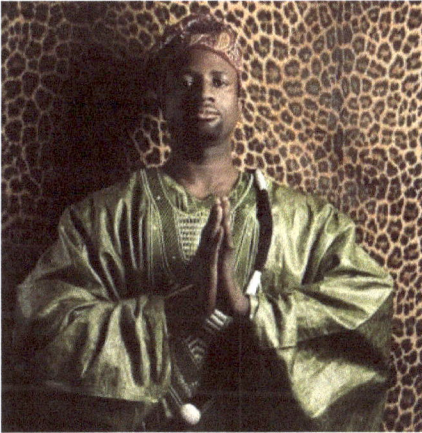

Standing

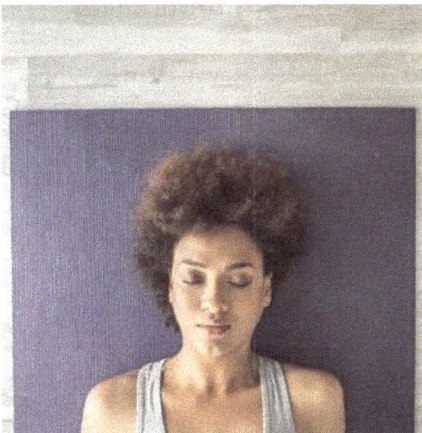

Laying down/flat

Finding Your Place

Now, let's find your sanctuary to practice this newfound skill. You must select a place for your meditation sessions. You'll want a location where you can spend time every day without interruption, as concentration is needed. While it doesn't need to be used solely for meditation, it is helpful to be at the same place for each sitting--especially as you try to create a new routine. The perfect spot can be wherever you decide; a favorite living room chair, in front of an altar if you have one, or maybe your bedroom, guest room wherever you find it to be most serene. Remember, it just needs to be somewhere that's comfortable and as quiet as possible. You don't have to have a separate room solely for mediation, as that maybe not is possible at the moment. The goal is to get someone you can be absorbed in your presence.

When you've found a place that feels good, you might choose to make the area special by having a favorite pillow or candle nearby. These things aren't necessary for meditation; they may simply enhance your experience and help bring you to a daily routine.

Not everybody has complete quiet time. You may have children or pets that need your attention, a noisy neighbor, or cars driving by. Try not to let this distract you too much. Meditation can be done even under the noisiest of circumstance try to disregard them and focus more on the inner connections. Please do not feel like you are at a disadvantage or that you won't get the results you desire. You may find the opposite is true. Having practiced meditation in a loud or raucous environment, you might soon discover that it's become natural for you to be at peace, no matter what is going on around you.

Preparation

Take some time out now to plan your meditation schedule for the week ahead. Ideally, you'll be able to sit during a morning hour, and if it can be the same hour each day, that's even better. Many people find that meditating just after they wake up is a great way to start their day. If you're not able to practice until later on in the afternoon or evening, or if you must sit at a different time each day, this is fine. It's far better to meditate anytime, than not at all.

As a best practice set aside 15 minutes each day. This will give you a couple of minutes on either side of your practice and allow for a sitting time of 5-10 minutes. With 10 minutes of meditation a day, you'll be able to see and feel results without putting too much pressure on yourself. Advanced practitioners will meditate 10, 20, 30, or more minutes per day. Pretty soon you'll understand how 10 minutes can be an easy routine to maintain.

After your sitting time is over, it's important to make sure that you're grounded. Sometimes meditating can bring you into higher realms and make it difficult to transition back to everyday reality. You may feel "floaty" and this can be a lovely feeling, but it means that you aren't securely grounded in your body and that is where you should be in daily life. There are many different techniques for grounding oneself, and you'll need to do some experimenting to come up with the practice that works best for you. You can try focusing your attention for a few moments on your connection to the earth, and where you are within it. Another way is to focus right below your navel area or at the base of your spine for a couple of minutes. You can also bring your awareness to your feet, and the feeling of your skin as it touches your floor, seat, or chair that you are sitting in.

Beginning Your Meditation Practice

It's that time you ready? Over the upcoming week, your job is to faithfully follow the meditation schedule you've created. You'll be sitting in meditation for 5 minutes every day and will undoubtedly have some interesting experiences. Try to pay attention to changes in the way you interpret and interact with the world outside of your meditation sessions. Do you feel calm? Anxious? Happy? Frustrated? There's no need to judge anything just be aware of those feelings & thoughts. This is simply an invitation to create greater self-awareness, which can help guide the way your practice evolves.

Let's get started:

1. Make sure you have on attire that is loose and does not restrict you or makes you uncomfortable.

2. Make sure to ensure minimum distractions by turning off alarms, ringers, televisions, etc.…

3. Prepare your meditation area as needed to your satisfaction. Candles, bells anything that sets the intentions of your practice.

4. Session Time: 5 minutes

When you are ready:

1. Take your position and begin to relax. Place your hand on your knees or thighs and open them up towards the ceiling, palms heavenward (ready to receive the blessings of the universe). Take a giant deep breath and let it out. Acknowledge that this is now your meditation time.

2. Now sit and begin to breathe more deeply, drawing the air in slowly and exhaling it at a comfortable rate. Make

sure your inhale is coming from your stomach and not your chest. Repeat this a few times.

1. Now simply sit and breathe. For the entire 5 minutes, just breathe. Make no judgment on what happens during this time. Most people will not be able to quiet their minds and may drift into thoughts about their to-do lists, what other people should or shouldn't have done, and even what's on the menu that day. Your mind may wander and that's perfectly okay. As soon as you realize your mind has led you somewhere else, release it, and breathe deeply. Do this every time your awareness leaves the present moment. If your mind comes up with something you cannot shake, write it down so you can get back to your awareness.

2. At the end of your session, take a couple of minutes to ground yourself. The act of grounding yourself is just returning to your present moment and once again be aware or conscious of the environment. I want you to feel floor underneath you, the bed or mattress, the couch. Think of how it feels on your body. Think of the sensation it gives your hips,

back arms etc.…think about the room you are in, wiggle your toes, and return to the present moment.

3. Take a moment and journal how you feel. Write your first experience down, what distractions did your experience? How many times were you able to catch your mind drifting during your session? What thoughts keep coming to you? What are those images that come to mind? I want to talk about these sessions with you at the end of the week so make sure you join our FB group. Post your first-week results in the FB group.

"It's up to you to break your family's generational curses!"

-Demetrius Irick

Breathing Techniques

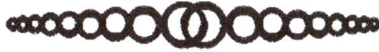

∞∞○○○○○ (○○) ○○○○○∞∞

Beginner Meditation

Week 2

 In the world of meditation it's so much we could cover but I would be remised if I didn't hammer home the foundation. This week we will dig a litter deeper into your breathing techniques. I will explore where you are currently and best practices for getting the most out of your session.

Have you noticed a shift in the ease or depth of your meditation experience? For the last seven days, you've been sitting for 5 minutes each session. Do you remember how difficult that was the first time? You may find that you're looking forward to your sessions now and that the time flies by quickly.

It's not the length of a sitting that creates long-term change, but the fact that you are taking the time and setting the intention that you are going to meditate and sit as long as you can. For this reason, you'll be continually reminded each week about the importance of practicing consistently. If you haven't been sitting in meditation every day, spend a few moments considering the obstacles that got in your way. If anything got in your way during your session log those in your journal.

Let's work on keeping your commitment to yourself & meditate with no distractions if possible. Those days that you missed a session…if you wanted to meditate, you could have made it work somehow. Don't let excuses rob you of a habit that will benefit every area of your life. You're the most important person in your world. Try not to be hard on yourself and simply pick up where you left off. To be of service to others, you have to keep yourself healthy and centered. Remember that every time you get on a plane and listen to the safety precautions presentation, the flight attendant urges you to put on your oxygen mask first. Think of meditation as a way to give yourself the very air you need. For those of us who have been meditating for years, that's exactly how it feels.

BREATH AWARENESS

The breath is one of the most important aspects of meditation. It acts as a point of focus and gives us a direct way to affect our sense of physical wellbeing. By simply taking deeper breaths, our physiology naturally responds; it relaxes and opens. If we become distracted by thoughts at any time in our meditation session, we can always return our attention to the breath. It's an ever-present, soothing rhythm. In both meditation and our daily lives, increasing our awareness of the feeling and sound of our breath can lead us to greater awareness and a calmer mind.

Before we continue, let's take a moment to consider how you're breathing right now. Gently feel how your belly and chest rise and fall with each inhale and exhale. Are your breaths shallow and fast? Or, are they slow and deep? Notice if your exhale is longer than the inhale, or vice-versa. No one answer is better than the other, these are simply things to watch and become aware of, even as you read through this lesson. Simply be aware or mindful.

The Breath

Breath sustains life. Every time we breathe, we choose to be apart of this thing we call life and it's a crazy cycle. We welcome in the air to oxygenate the nearly 30 trillions cells in our body and send out the carbon dioxide to be recycled after it we've used it. The breathing process is the inhale and exhale. There is a brief moment of space between each breath on the inhale and exhale which completes the cycle of breathing.

When taking in the air it provides our body with the essential substance we need to sustain this life we live. With each inhale we draw into ourselves a vital aspect of life; through inhaling we attract, invite, allow, and receive. In this way, we open up ourselves to all that life has to offer. We open ourselves up to the universe and the many blessings it has for everyone.

All of us know how good it feels to step off an airplane or out of a smoky room and take our first big breath of fresh air. The whole world opens up again. We immediately feel reinvigorated. When we're in an atmosphere that feels negative for any reason--from a cigarette smoke-filled room to an angry person yelling harsh words, we tend to shut down our inhale and don't realize we do it.

Just for a minute, without changing anything yet, place some attention on the way you're inhaling right now. Pay attention to where your breathing originates…are you breathing from your chest or stomach? Start taking bigger, deeper breaths, still focusing only on your inhale. How does your body feel when you breathe in fully, filling your lungs with air? Notice the experience in your whole body--chest, belly, arms, and legs, head. Pay attention to the muscles as they relax because of the air traveling throughout the body. What are the physical sensations you are feeling right now? Are there any nonphysical sensations or thoughts that come to mind? I want you to sit here for a minute. I want you to tune into this for several minutes. I need you to understand the messages your body tells you through the aches, pain, and thoughts that occur. What do you feel? What thoughts come to mind? Continue the deep breathing in and out...feel your being feel rejuvenated.

1. The Exhale: Releasing and Radiating

Exhaling is the way our body releases air we've used and offers it to other forms of life like plants. Both literally and symbolically, the process of breathing out is a manner of letting go. We release carbon dioxide, and through this very action, lymph fluid gets pumped through bodies and our muscles relax. This, the letting go, is an essential and helpful part of life.

You've probably heard the expression "breathed a sigh of relief." That's the way it feels to exhale. It's taking all the tension that is inside of us, and all the tension that builds from inhaling and letting it all disappear. There's a feeling of satisfaction when we breathe out. Our needs have been met and we can rest.

Exhaling can also be thought of as an opportunity to radiate well wishes out into the universe. It can be a way of sending our intentions out to find their manifestation. Our society already understands this. Just remember the last birthday party you went to the birthday girl or boy "makes a wish" just before blowing out the candles.

Take a minute to become aware of your breath as you exhale. How does your body feel when you let the air out of your lungs? Are there any non-physical sensations associated with this? Notice the experience in your whole body--chest, belly, arms, and legs, head. Tune into this for several minutes.

2. The Space Between the Breath: Stillness
Now that you've explored the inhale and the exhale, it's time to address the more passive part of the breathing cycle: the space between the breath. This occurs both at the point just before inhalation and at the point just before exhalation. It is also often described as the moment when you are neither

inhaling nor exhaling. Without holding air in or forcing it out, simply take note of this moment when no air is flowing in either direction. Concentrate on this for a few breath cycles. There's deep peace, stillness. See if you can feel it. Within this space exists pure possibility. When your focus is brought here, the space between the breath naturally expands and both the inhale and the exhale organically deepen. It's an almost magical way of changing your rate of breath and helping your body to relax.

Breathing Cycle

All these parts of breathing make up the breath cycle. Take some time now to explore the full cycle in its entirety. Pay attention to all the different parts--the inhale, the exhale, and the two spaces between the breath, bringing consciousness to each as you go along. Pay attention to the different parts that feel concerning each other. Tune in to the way they complement one another. Perhaps there's a sense of fulfillment, completion, as you move from beginning to end. Perhaps you feel peace at how natural and inevitable this process is.

Breathing Practices

Now that you understand the breath cycle and how significant a role breathing plays in meditation, do your best to apply what you know as a means to enhance your practice. Each distracting thought is a great opportunity to return awareness to your breathing and reconnect with the ever-present flow of air being brought in and released back out.

Meditation for Relaxation

Several very simple breathing practices are done to aid in stress reduction and general relaxation. Some of them may originate with an ancient meditation tradition and the meditator may invent others to have an effective customized program.

Here's an example of a simple breathing meditation:
First, through your nose, take a nice, long breath. Slowly. Deeply. Let it out your mouth. If you care to, let out a nice long sigh to release any tension you may have. Making an

audible "Ahhhh" sound while exhaling can help relax the tenser body parts.

Next, focus your attention on the emptiness of your lungs. Wait until your lungs feel "ready" to fill with air again. Through your nose again, inhale slowly, filling your lungs to their greatest capacity. When you feel almost ready to burst, let out a nice "Ahhhhhh" on the exhale. Repeat three times. (It's important to try and not be embarrassed when exhaling, be loud with your "Ahhhhhhh" if it feels right)

Another simple technique involves paying attention to the breath at the point of entry and exit through the nostrils. The very sensation of the breath entering and leaving the nostrils is used as the point of focus for the entire sitting. Simple adaptations can be made to meditations such as this.

For example, you might slow your breath specifically on the exhale, so that breathing out takes twice as long as breathing in. Another change might be to try removing the space between the breaths so that there is only constant flow and rhythm.

5 Power Of Breathing Technique

The number five is a powerful number it's not ordinary. The number daily surrounds us as humans and some of us don't marvel in its subtle strength. It's no coincidence; the human body has five fingers on each hand and five toes on each foot. It's no coincidence that we have five senses: sight, smell, taste, touch, and hearing and thus five sensory organs: eyes, nose, tongue, skin, and ears.

The "5-5-5: Core Breathing" is an easy, relaxing breath technique that can be practiced anywhere. At first, the effects of this exercise may be subtle, but its effects compound over time with repetition and practice helps your practice.

In this chapter, I will introduce the power of 5 breathing technique. It's simple and easy to use to keep you focused, and grounded.

5-5-5 Breathing Core Steps:

1. Rest your tongue lightly along the roof of your mouth. Allow it to rest there throughout the exercise.

2. Exhale completely before you start a new cycle of breath.

3. Close your mouth; inhale quietly through your nose as you count to five. Let your belly and chest fill up with breath.

4. Pause. Hold your breath for a count of five.

5. Exhale completely through your mouth, making a 'whoosh' sound, as you count to **five again.** Let your belly and chest release all it's air pushing out all of the air from your belly.

- Steps 3-5 make one full breath cycle. Repeat these steps for a total of five rounds. Try practicing this **twice daily,** to start, working yourself to five times per day.

Tips:

- Inhale quietly through your nose and exhale audibly through your mouth.
- Keep your tongue relaxed on the roof of your mouth throughout.
- If you have trouble holding your breath, consider speeding up your count.
- After a month or so of practice, you may extend your breath cycles. Keep working up to longer holds and exhales, as is comfortable for you. Exhales are cooling, calming, and invigorating!
- Lightheadedness is a normal side effect when you begin to practice. Continue to focus and remain calm until it passes. If it does not pass, return to your normal breathing pattern.

Alternate Nostril Breathing

Another technique primarily involves the nostrils. Most of us are used to breathing in and out of both nostrils at the same time.

In order to get an optimal amount of oxygen to the brain and to get both sides of the brain fully functioning, you can practice a technique known as Alternate Nostril Breathing. This style of breathing can increase creativity and verbal skills, and also improve mental stamina.

Take your hand and gently pinch closed your left nostril. Now breathe in and out your right nostril for three complete breaths.

Now change sides by closing your right nostril and breathing through your left nostril for three complete breaths.

Repeat on each side three times.

Breathing from the Diaphragm

Breathing from the diaphragm can sometimes be a part of the pranayama practice and it is often recommended in many other meditative exercises. Your meditation sitting can become easier and more profound simply from learning how to breathe this way.

Many of us have developed a lifelong habit of breathing into our chests, which is by nature a very shallow way of breathing. Breathing from the diaphragm, however, engages the diaphragm muscles that are located lower in our bodies. The result is calmer, deeper breaths. The heart becomes energized and the nervous system is soothed.

Learning how to breathe this new way can take some time. Many of us are so used to breathing with our upper chest that we find it a challenge to breathe using this alternate muscle group.

The key to breathing from the diaphragm is in understanding exactly where it's located. The diaphragm is shaped like an upside-down dome and sits just below the bottom of the rib cage, stretching the full horizontal width of the body. When inhaling from the diaphragm, the diaphragm muscle contracts, pulling downward and slightly flaring out the ribs. The bottoms of the lungs are pulled down and bring in the air. With exhaling, the upper abdomen just below the breastbone inverts slightly to fully express the air. If you're doing this correctly, you'll find that there's almost no motion in your lower abdomen or upper chest as you breathe.

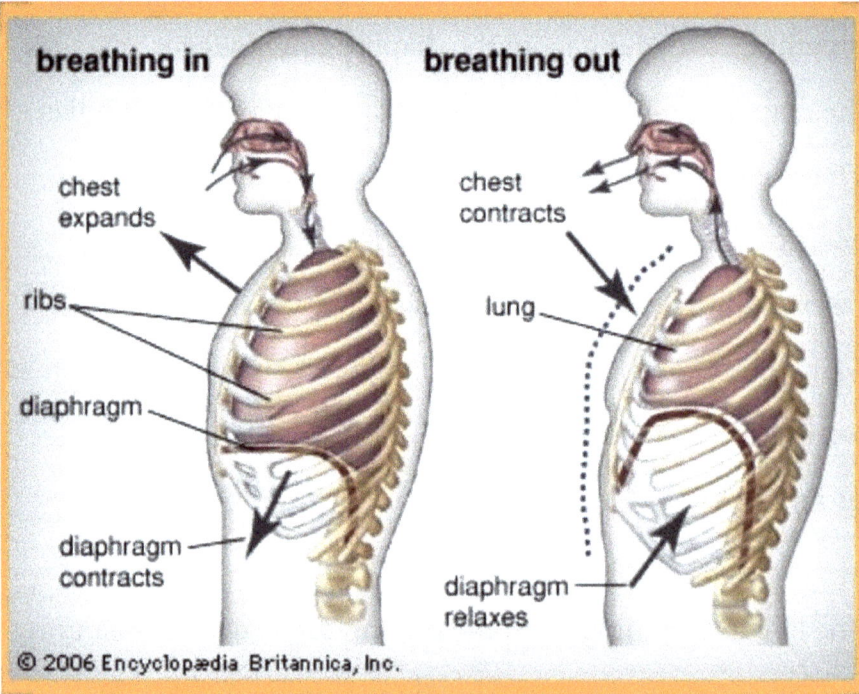

breathing in

chest expands

ribs

diaphragm

diaphragm contracts

breathing out

chest contracts

lung

diaphragm relaxes

© 2006 Encyclopædia Britannica, Inc.

It's that time again to schedule your meditation practice for the week ahead. If you haven't been sitting each day despite having the time blocked out in your calendar, see if you might find a time of day that makes it easier for you to follow through. Perhaps you've already established a set routine of meditating at a particular time each day, and maybe you've been doing this consistently. If this is the case, keep on going--you're on the right track.

For this week's practice, we're going to show you how to begin breathing with your diaphragm, as it will prove helpful in your ongoing experience with meditation. Please be patient with yourself here. This is a different way of moving your body then you're probably used to. When you're doing it correctly, you'll know. You'll be able to feel the difference in your body and it's even possible you may feel a little sore.

The following is a step-by-step guide. You may wish to print out this lesson and carry it with you into your sittings.

BREATHING FROM THE DIAPHRAGM MEDITATION

Demetrius Irick

Let's get started:

1. Make sure you have on attire that is loose and does not restrict you or makes you uncomfortable.

2. Make sure to ensure minimum distractions by turning off alarms, ringers, televisions, etc.…

3. Prepare your meditation area as needed to your satisfaction. Candles, bells anything that sets the intentions of your practice.

4. Session Time: 5 minutes

When you are ready:

1. Take your position and begin to relax. Place your hand on your knees or thighs and open them up towards the ceiling, palms heavenward (ready to receive the blessings of the universe). Take a giant deep breath and let it out. Acknowledge that this is now your meditation time.

2. Now sit and begin to breathe more deeply, drawing the air in slowly and exhaling it at a comfortable rate. Make sure your inhale is coming from your stomach and not your chest. Repeat this a few times.

3. Place your right hand over your chest in the area of your heart. Place your left hand over your abdomen. Inhale through your nose and allow your abdomen to rise. Continue slowly inhaling until your chest cavity is filled with air. You may feel your belly moving out and away from your lower spine. Do this slowly.

4. Now exhale through the nose. Allow your abdomen to release the air. As you do this, feel your belly pulling in and your muscles tighten toward your lower spine.

5. Continue practicing steps 3 and 4 throughout your sitting. If your mind begins to wander, simply bring your attention back to your breathing. Remember that your upper chest and lower abdomen do not move very much (or even at all) when you're breathing from your diaphragm.

6. At the end of your session, take a couple of minutes to ground yourself. The act of grounding yourself is just returning to your present moment. I want you to feel the floor underneath you, the bed or mattress, the couch. Think of how it feels on your body. Think of the sensation it gives your hips,

back arms etc....think about the room you are in, wiggle your toes, and return to the present moment.

7. Take a moment and journal how you feel. Write your first experience down, what distractions did your experience? How many times were you able to catch your mind drifting during your session? What thoughts keep coming to you? What are those images that come to mind? I want to talk about these sessions with you at the end of the week so make sure you join our FB group. Post this week's results in the FB group.

"Be as the sand at the bottom of the ocean ready to move at all times...never avoiding it but agile in it's essence of what it's purpose is. When you are able to do this...it doesn't matter whether its raining, storming, or sunshine...you will be grounded in your essence!"

-Demetrius Irick

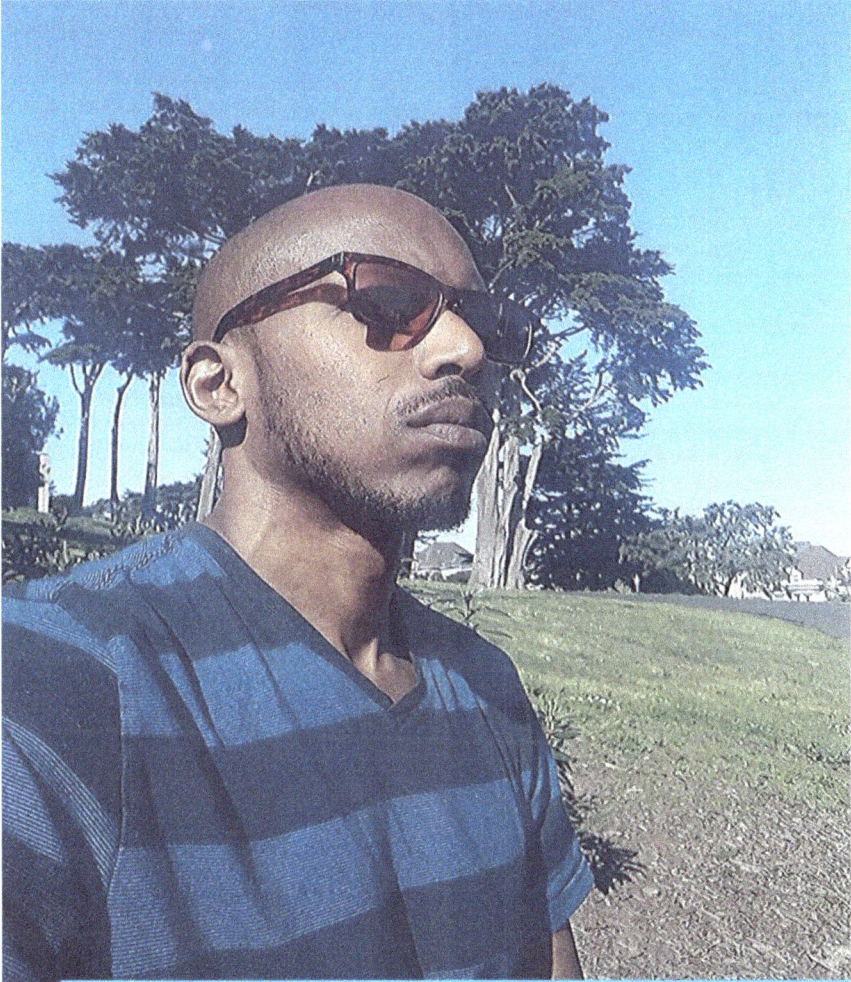

FRSH SUN x FRSH AIR x FRSH WATER

Mindfulness

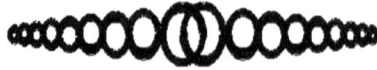

Beginner Meditation

Week 3

All right, week three congrats! Now that you have been meditating for another week, there is no doubt that you will have some observable preferences; as such you'll have to reflect a bit on your experience. You may have discovered that the process got easier as the days progressed, or you may have discovered that your mind wonders more than you realized. You may have discovered that you had a lot more energy throughout the week or felt less anxious. Hey, maybe your butt, legs, and thighs are a little sore from sitting in new positions. One thing is for sure every person's experience will be unique, both in these first weeks and after years of practicing there are no wrong or right ways only what feels good for you.

Remember, the most important component of helpful meditation practice is that you do it regularly. It is called a meditation practice or a reason. I hope you were able to sit for a little practice each day this week. Remember the more you continue, you'll begin to look forward to your meditation time each day as an opportunity to be nurtured, calmed, and refreshed.

The Journey of quieting the MIND

We are not our thoughts we are the origin of those thoughts. You ever did something and then asked yourself " Why did I do that?" We have all whether conscious or not witnessed the power of the mind to create drama in our lives. It's up to us to put into our minds and body things that create wellness and peace. We should invest in our lives with a sense of determination & focus to generate healthy lifestyle habits. That's ultimately what you are doing now…being conscious to invest in your inner peace.

Demetrius Irick

I am sure you have heard the saying " You are what you eat!" The same is true with the things we put into our minds and spirit. We must put things that inspire us, encourages us to want to do better and be better people in life.

The power of the mind is simply amazing. It is programmed in a way of infinite thoughts, which may not be easily suppressed but can be surpassed. What are the chances of someone with this thought process winning? " I don't think I can do it!" verses, "There must be a way for me to get it done!" The perception is the key...

I heard this parable and it stuck with me. There was a man that looked out of his house and found a man digging in his garbage for food. He said to himself...God, I am thankful I am not in that position; I wish this man the best. The man that went through the garbage went about his way and saw a man being arrested for stealing a sandwich out of a local gas station. He said, Thank you, God, that I am not in that position, I wish him the best. As the man was sitting in the back of the cop car being sent to jail, he saw a young man race across the street getting hit by a car, blood everywhere and paralyzed from the waist down, he said to himself, Thank you, God, that I am not in that position, I wish him well. The paralyzed guy lay in his hospital bed and wept at the thought of him not being able to walk again. His nurse entered as he wept and asked him was, he okay? The man explained his pain and the nurse responded, Thank God you are not in the place the man was that was in this bed before you. The man looked as the nurse pointed to the room across from him labeled coroner office! Praise Our Creator for the progress and where you are...your viewpoint can determine if you will crawl under a rock or reach for the sky! Don't compare your progress to anyone else. It's up to you to do the work and be patient with yourself because this is a journey, not a speed race.

What matters is our perspective of every situation. Our perspective will always have a positive or negative impact on our minds. When we see something that is scary, it is in human nature to develop the fear of the unknown, but it takes a conscious mind to identify and look beyond the fear. It takes perseverance and dedication to this goal you have established...keep practicing, be completed conquer the fear that dwells within. Conquer the part of you that fights when you try to do something good for your life. Fight for yourself...fight to be better than you were the day before.

When we meditate, we are aware of the thoughts in our mind... and we realize how fast the thoughts go from one extreme to the other. With practice, we can make it a little easier to still our mind from always racing. In reality, the thoughts will always be there they are just not as loud. They retreat to being in the background and not demanding so much attention. It's at this point when we begin to choose positive thoughts from this sense of peace, stillness, and awareness. Meditation increases our strength and gives us mental fortitude to push past self-limiting thoughts. It helps us gain control over our lives and enables focus, which is a powerful tool and a great habit to obtain.

The mind will wander as it has since humans were created. Even when you gain more discipline and better control your mind it will still wander.

We like to call it the "Monkey Mind", the racing of thoughts at the speed of light. Ever since humans first began meditating, we have needed to develop strategies for dealing with the monkey mind. This is because once we step back from our everyday activities and sit in silence; we can finally hear the insanity and frantic pace of our thoughts. Most strategies for taming the monkey mind involve deliberately directing our attention to a specific thing. Many meditators, for example, focus on their breathing. Breathing is one of the most basic methods for quieting and training the mind. The practice involves placing simple awareness of the inhale and the exhale. Breathe in. Breathe out. Breathe in. Breathe out. Breathe in. Breathe out. It's a steady, relaxing rhythm and is perfect for calming mental chatter.

Demetrius Irick

Mental Awareness

The more you practice, the easier it becomes to be aware of when your mind wonders and the ability to return to your breathe or focus point. Don't ever think meditation is about stopping your thoughts. It's your mind's job to think. That's simply what it does. There's nothing good or bad about this. It's whether you choose to feed the thoughts that determine whether you (and sometimes those you affect) will have pleasant or unpleasant experiences as a result. The thoughts themselves just come and they go. There is a term for this called, "rise and fall away." And this is exactly what your thoughts, and even your feelings, do: arise and fall away.

There is one technique called "Naming", where you just assign a name to each thought (and feeling) that arises. This is suggested as a way of attending to each thought without getting lost in it. The process goes something like this: Let's say you're sitting in meditation and there is a thought that emerges about how much work needs to get done before the end of the day. According to this method, you might name that thought as "work", "worry," "anxiety," or "anticipation," etc. If you were to think about an ex-boyfriend or girlfriend you're missing, you might label that thought as "love," "longing," or another appropriate term. After each time you name the thought in this fashion, you return awareness to your breathing. The more you do this you will find that the distraction seems to lessen throughout your practice.

Mindfulness

Through meditation and gaining awareness of our thoughts, we begin to understand a term called "mindfulness." This means bringing consciousness into any and every experience. When we are mindful, we are not jumping around with our monkey minds, judging this and qualifying that; we are open, aware, and entirely present.

Practicing mindfulness can be such joy and brings about healing at times. Imagine that after you come home from a very stressful day at work you find that your dog figured out how to get out of his cage and have run rampant throughout the house damaging furniture, using the bathroom and tearing up papers all over the house. Now, if you react from an unconscious place you may lash out at the dog. If you respond in mindfulness you simply take a deep breath, see what needs to be done to fix the problem, and fix it. We know that the dog has made a mess and that we are frustrated by the actions of the dog. The truth of the matter is that regardless of your anger the mess has to be cleaned and you have to do it. So maybe after cleaning up or prior depending on your state of mind you need to take a walk around the block before you strangle the dog? (Smile)

The beauty is that you decided on how you were going to deal with the situation instead of reacting from your emotional state…you responded mindfully about your next move. You made a conscious choice in alignment with the peace you desired and needed. You were MINDFUL!!!!

Continuing Your Meditation Practice

Take some time now to schedule your daily meditation time for the week ahead. Remember to give yourself about five minutes extra for getting prepared and for then grounding yourself after the meditation.

This week we're going to practice a very simple meditation that can be used any time to begin a session. It's a very easy way to clear your mind of distracting thoughts and move into a steady stream of awareness. The following is a step-by-step guide for this technique. You may wish to print out this lesson and carry it with you into your sittings.

Demetrius Irick

MINDFULNESS MEDITATION

Let's get started:

1. Make sure you have on attire that is loose and does not restrict you or makes you uncomfortable.

2. Make sure to ensure minimum distractions by turning off alarms, ringers, televisions, etc.…

3. Prepare your meditation area as needed to your satisfaction. Candles, bells anything that sets the intentions of your practice.

4. Session Time: 10 minutes

When you are ready:

1. Take your position and begin to relax. Place your hand on your knees or thighs and open them up towards the ceiling, palms heavenward (ready to receive the blessings of the universe). Take a giant deep breath and let it out. Acknowledge that this is now your meditation time.

2. Now sit and begin to breathe more deeply, drawing the air in slowly and exhaling it at a comfortable rate. Make sure

your inhale is coming from your stomach and not your chest. Repeat this a few times.

3. As you inhale, begin to pay attention to your body starting at the crown of your head. Put all your attention there and gradually move down your body until you reach your feet. Each part of your body pay attention to any tension, stress, anxiety, uneasiness, or unrest. Repeat this process 5 times. For each body part, you put your attention to spend 10-15 seconds on each part. Get into it feel it…get in tune with your body.

4. When you are ready, breath out naturally and take a few deep breathes, drawing in the air slowly and exhaling it at a comfortable rate.

5. At the end of your session, take a couple of minutes to ground yourself. The act of grounding yourself is just returning to your present moment and once again be conscious of the environment. Pay close attention to the floor underneath you, the bed or mattress, the couch. Think of how it feels on your body. Think of the sensation it gives your hips,

back arms etc.…think about the room you are in, wiggle your toes, and return to the present moment.

6. Take a moment and journal how you feel. Write your first experience down, what distractions did your experience? How many times were you able to catch your mind drifting during your session? What thoughts keep coming to you? What are those images that come to mind? I want to talk about these sessions with you at the end of the week so make sure you join our FB group. Post this week's results in the FB group.

"The storms of life will knock on your door...it's how well you prepare for them that will determine how devastating it's impact will be!"

-Demetrius Irick

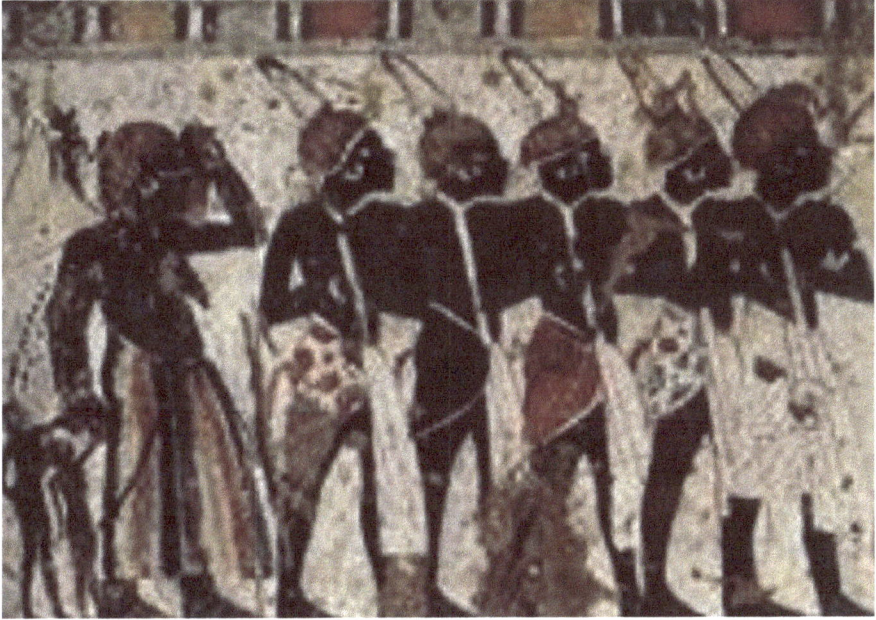

"The moment we come back to our roots and understand who we are there is an awakening in the depth of our soul that yearns to be blessings to all we come in contact with."

-Demetrius Irick

Demetrius Irick

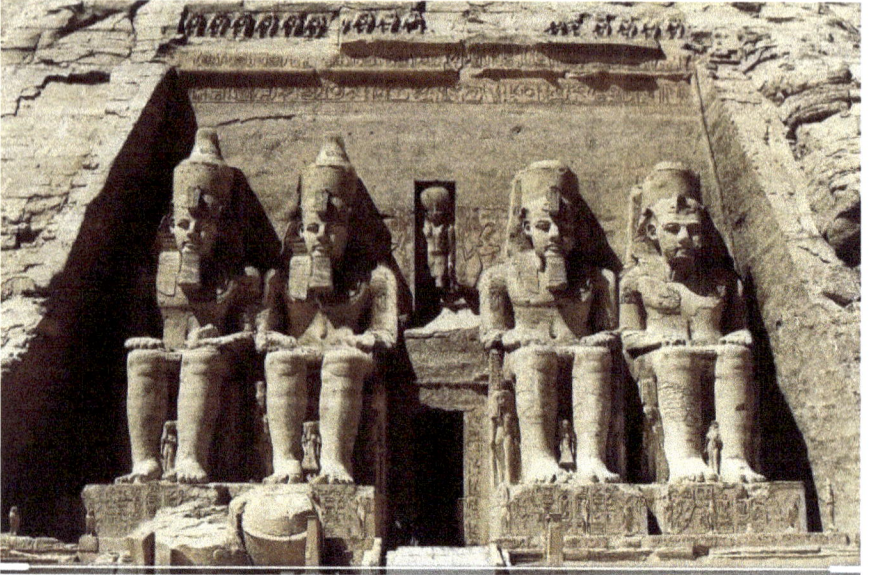

"Our Ancestor's craved statues of themselves in the mountains so you wouldn't forget your heritage. They painted themselves in specific colors so the world would know who and what they looked like when they left this world yet with all of the evidence and proof the children are blind."

D. Irick.

Meditation Through Sight and Scent

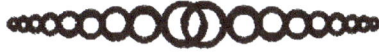

<u>Beginner Meditation</u>

<u>Week 4</u>

Did you clear out any obstacles or excuses that were in the way before? I am hopeful that you found your way around anything that prevented you from reaching your goals. Hopefully, you've built a steady practice that you can look forward to each day. Remember, your meditation time is a gift for yourself. It's your little piece of joy, a reward to your inner being for doing the self-healing work.

EXPLORING MEDITATION THROUGH SIGHTS & SCENTS
The beauty that meditation provides is it allows us the ability to reach out of the realm of sensation and into a state of pure existence, pure awareness. There will be times when the dog is barking, the phone rings unexpectedly, a spouse or loved one interrupts you or make too much noise but instead of

getting angry or agitated, we can continue peacefully aware and judgment-free in our meditative state

.

As humans, we have five core physical senses: sight, scent, hearing, touch, and taste. Our senses can help us draw valuable information and navigate through our environment. It's amazing how our body and mind is hardwired. There are smells and scents we receive from our sense of smell that triggers memories…activating the part of our brain to travel through time. There is the sight of a snake or bear, that triggers fear and our body sends chemicals to our physical body, which in turn can affect the way we process information or think. There are certain songs we hear that bring joy, or pain to our mental and physical bodies. Again, it's amazing how our body uses the senses to interact in this physical world.

This knowledge about the power of sensory input is what fields like aromatherapy (literally, "aromatherapy") are based upon. They specialize in using our sense of smell to enact an emotional state of relaxation.

Our ancestors knew that the mind needed something to keep us focus at times. They understood that on occasion to keep us focused on a sensation or to minimize getting distracted by our passing thoughts our sense of smell can be used. They understood that short inspirational affirmations, or mantras, could often be repeated many times during one's meditation as well to keep focused. During some of the sessions, drums were used to keep the practitioner's mind focused on the rhythm, and some burned incense to affect their mind through scent.

Over the next week, we'll learn more about techniques like this, and determine what works best for you and your practice. The beauty of creation and humans is that we are all different and what works for me may not work for you but given these options, you will have the education to make the best decision for you!

This week we're exploring meditation through techniques involving two senses: sight and scent.

Sight

Birds and humans use vision as our primary sense. Many animals such as cats & dogs interpret the world through smell first, then hearing, then sight. We will start with sight. During this technique, we will leave our eyes open and direct all of our attention to a particular object that we have in front of us. I suggest a candle flame and or the smoke from burning incense. These have given me trance-like states and sensations that sweep me up during my sessions.

1. Visualizations:

When you can create a picture, vision, or image in your mind you can visualize. Visualizations in meditation can be huge…and so many messages come to those that can do this. Unfortunately, everyone doesn't have this and that's cool as well. I struggle with visualization.

Someone that can close their eyes and envision being on a spacecraft headed to the moon, feel the pressure as their feet touch the moon, or picking up a rock on Mars…with vivid details is a power some wished they had.

There are some techniques where you visualize and see family members that have passed on and you receive messages from them either from an image or a feeling in your body. These are used to help you on your journey in life.

Scent

Our ancestors knew the sense of smell activates emotions, certain states of awareness, and thus they used different incenses and smells to meditate. Throughout the practice, you will find that certain fragrances can relax the mind more so than others. It's funny but our brain makes an immediate connection with certain scents. This is one reason it is helpful to use the same kind of incense for every sitting when you determine the ones that work for you. The more you work with those scents throughout your life and day if you smell those scents it takes you mentally in a meditative state even if at the time you are not meditating…Cool Right!

Demetrius Irick

There are many different incense fragrances. Some favorites are dragon blood and sage, lavender, nag champa, fruit scents, fresh linen etc. It doesn't matter what you decide but I suggest something fresh, and that appeals to your inner body sensations when you smell it.

This week, I want you to work daily with sight and smell meditations. I would like you to use candles or incense with your practice. I want you to compare the past week's meditations against this week. I want you to determine if your mind seems to gravitate to a certain smell or does the flame help to ease your stress and anxiety. Does the flame allow your mind to be at peace? Ideally, it will allow your mind to flow into a peaceful state more easily. However, you may find that this is more difficult with your eyes open than with your eyes closed. Here again, there is no right or wrong response. You'll simply want to be aware of how effective this method is for you personally. Following is a step-by-step guide to the method you'll be using. You may wish to print out this lesson and carry it with you into your sittings.

Determine what your focal point will be. Choose an item that feels most appropriate and calming for you. To remind you of some objects commonly used by meditators, you could decide to work with an image of a deity, a lit candle or incense, an object from nature, or anything else you personally select. What's important is that the item allows your mind to focus, rather than encouraging it to drift. Photos of family or loved ones are often not recommended, as they can stir up emotions and memories that would interfere with the process.

FOCUSED MEDITATION

Before you begin:

1. Make sure you have on attire that is loose and does not restrict you or makes you uncomfortable.

2. Make sure to ensure minimum distractions by turning off alarms, ringers, televisions, etc....

3. Prepare your meditation area as needed to your satisfaction. Candles, bells anything that sets the intentions of your practice.

4. Session Time: 10 minutes

When you are ready:

1. Once you've selected your object, approach your meditation area, and place this object a few feet in front of where you'll be sitting. If you've been meditating while lying on a bed because you cannot physically sit, try to lie on one side for this particular practice session, and place the chosen object in a safe place in your line of sight. Since you'll be meditating with your eyes open, you'll want to be able to see the object from where you're seated or lying, without having to tilt your head too far up or down.

2. Take your position and begin to relax. Place your hand on your knees or thighs and open them up towards the ceiling, palms heavenward (ready to receive the blessings of the universe). Take a giant deep breath and let it out. Acknowledge that this is now your meditation time.

3. Now sit and begin to breathe more deeply, drawing the air in slowly and exhaling it at a comfortable rate. Make sure your inhale is coming from your stomach and not your chest. Repeat this a few times.

4. With your eyes open, allow your eyelids to rest about a third of the way closed. You'll want to hold a soft gaze that is slightly out of focus and place your attention on the item you've chosen. As you do this, it is okay to blink softly and naturally.

5. Now simply sit and breathe. For the entire length of your session, just breathe and focus on your item. Make no judgment on what happens. Your mind may wander and that's perfectly okay. As soon as you realize your mind has led you somewhere else, release it, and breathe deeply. Do this every time your awareness leaves the object and the present moment. Remember to allow your gaze to be soft and your eyes to rest naturally.

6. At the end of your session, take a couple of minutes to ground yourself. The act of grounding yourself is just returning to your present moment and once again be conscious of the environment. I want you to pay attention to the floor underneath you, the bed or mattress, the couch. Think of how it feels on your body. Think of the sensation it

gives your hips, back arms etc....think about the room you are in, wiggle your toes, and return to the present moment.

7. Take a moment and journal how you feel. Write your first experience down, what distractions did your experience? How many times were you able to catch your mind drifting during your session? What thoughts keep coming to you? What are those images that come to mind? I want to talk about these sessions with you at the end of the week so make sure you join our FB group. Post this week's results in the FB group.

"You don't have a chance at being successful unless you tame your inner fears that causes you to sabotage your goals!"

-Demetrius Irick

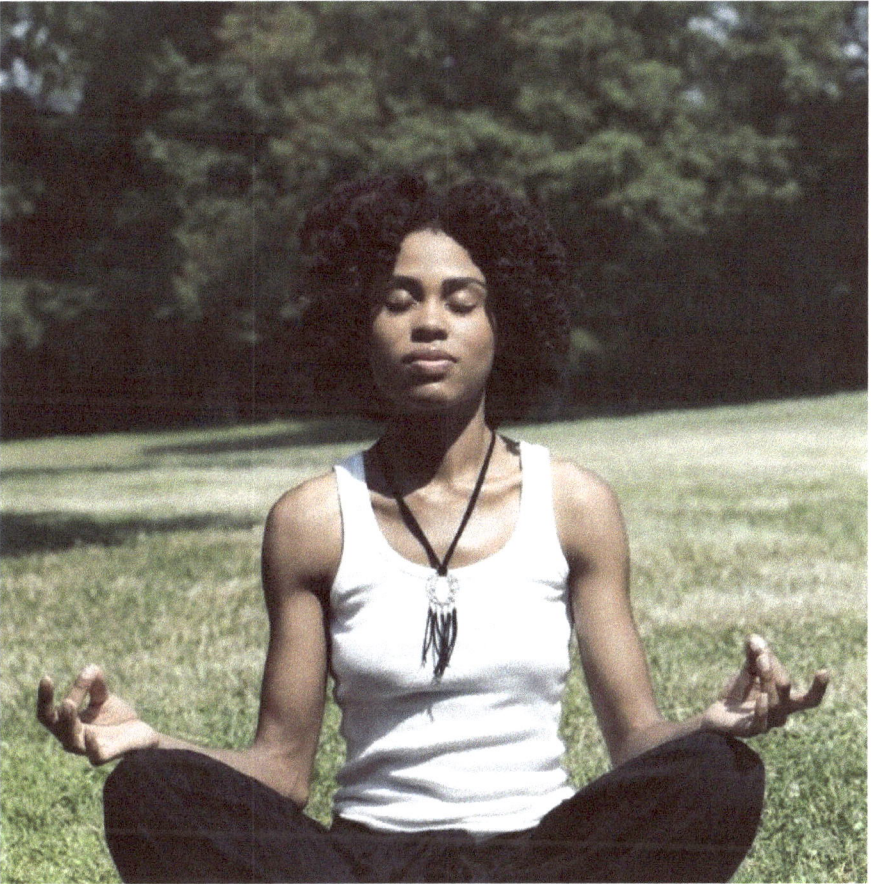

"Meditation is an investment in present & future self. Do you believe that your are worth the investment?"

-Demetrius Irick

Meditation Through Words (Mantras)

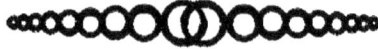

Beginner Meditation

Week 5

Mantra Meditation

It's time to celebrate yourself, you've been meditating for one whole month and we're at the halfway point. Let's take some time to evaluate where you are thus far.

1.) Meditation place. So, analyze your spot is it safe?

Have you avoided being interrupted during your sessions? How's has that worked for you? If not, explore some alternative places until you find one that works.

2.) Sitting Positions. Remember that first week of sitting and the aches and pains it caused you? Has it gotten easier to sit up straight? Now, is a good time to make adjustments as needed with your sitting positions.

3.) Clothing. Are you wearing the right things for extended sitting? Your clothing should be so comfortable that you don't notice it during your session.

4.) Time. Have you been allowing enough time during and around your session to ensure its enough time allowing you to be effective in your inner work?

5.) Routine. Have you been able to build a routine around your meditation practice? Is morning meditation best for your lifestyle or some other time?

6.) Improvement. Take a minute and just reflect on your month. What adjustments would you like to make? Now, is a great time to just plan out changes for the next few weeks. Remember, everything we are doing is about you.

Demetrius Irick

(MANTRAS & CHANTING)

Since the beginning of time, our ancestors knew about the power of sound and the effects it has on one's internal wellbeing. In meditation, words are used to focus the mind, while deepening and heightening the meditative experience. Now, we are about to explore a few common mantras that we will work on this week.

Mantras

There is no general or conventional definition of the word 'mantra' as it varies from culture and languages. However, the term "mantra" can refer to any commonly repeated word or phrase. They are sacred syllables, words, and utterances that have spiritual or psychological leadings/power. Sometimes they can form a structure or specific meaning and sometimes they don't. The structure composed of various elements that drive humans into actions such as truth, peace, love, knowledge, and light.

Originally, however, mantras were used in African Spirituality, and eventually Eastern religious practices such as Buddhism and Hinduism. A mantra involved specific words or syllables from the ancient (Sanskrit language) that were used as a formula for activating higher states of awareness. The meditator would repeat the mantra over and over to quiet their mind and prepare their energy for communion with the Source.

Sanskrit has been described as a language of physics, meaning that the specific tones and vibrations of the words, when spoken, have an immediate effect on the physical body. For example, the Sanskrit syllable Om (pronounced "Aum") expresses the sound, or vibration, of pure consciousness, pure energy. When spoken as a mantra, an individual call his or her cells into resonance with this essential state of being. The meditative experience can become quite deep and restorative simply from repeating this one sound several times.

Mantras can be short, as in the syllable Om, or a few sentences long as in the Gayatri Mantra. The Gayatri Mantra is considered to be the oldest and most transformative of all the Ancient Eastern mantras. For some people, though, saying a mantra in a foreign language isn't particularly helpful and they find greater benefit from using one of their makings. You can create a mantra that's as simple as "love" or "peace." Or, you may use a short sentence such as, "I am," or "All is well." Whichever is of greatest help in focusing your mind is the one to be used. The mantra can be said aloud or silently.

The chanting can be seen as a mystical experience as the sounds, singing, meditation makes your body a temple or divine instrument through which a particular level of connection is achieved. It mostly speeds up by the right mindset of the practitioner. Your intentions will determine the type of chants you should use.

This makes it important to know the reason you want to perform it. You should also understand the power of sound as it connects meaning to the subconscious thereby generating a focus towards maintaining chats with divinity. It is advisable to secure a quiet spot for the chant just to avoid or overlook all forms of distractions. At this level, phone calls, television, or other external sound notifications may not be necessary. You can as well add incense or candle to the spot where you want to chant just to help you maintain a reasonable magnitude of focus.

Meditation Beads

Meditation beads can be used in meditation to track the number of times a mantra is spoken. This is done in a way similar to how Catholics count prayers using rosary beads. In Buddhist and Hindu practices, the meditation beads used are called Mala beads. Simply, these are 108 beads strung in a circle. When you have decided to use the mantra during meditation, the practitioner must clarify their intention to know the kind of mala beads to use. Once you've decided on the beads, you must find a comfortable place and sit appropriately in a cross-legged position. While maintaining the sitting position, you must observe the speed of your mind and your natural deep breaths. This breath will begin to channel you towards achieving a focus in your mind and on the mantra.

You will also have to hang the mala beads in the finger of either of your hands, whichever you prefer to be comfortable. It is also important to place your thumb on the head bead before chanting your desires and at the end of each mantra after highlighting your wishes comfortably, you will have to shift the bead from your thumb to a side before you start with the next round and can only stop until you have counts, 7, 21, 27, or 108 depending on the time and chanting length you've decided to reach.

This process of prayer will continue until you are convinced in your mind that the divine has granted your desires. Mala is more of a meditative tool used to reach the path of spiritual endeavor. There is no definite or good mantra as everything to be used can be as simple as possible depending on your desire. The mala beads are usually 7-10mm in size and their shape is not too heavy so it can be used easily during prayers. They are usually made with lotus seed beads, Bodhi seeds, and wood. Their properties and color can be extracted from black onyx, rose quartz, jade, and turquoise. Invariably all mala beads can be worn as a necklace or wrapped bracelets by the practitioner and many of them can easily wear it back whenever they have completed their prayers just to remind them of their next scheduled time of prayer. Remember that whichever mala beads you've decided to use for your chants, you would hold the beads in your left hand and slide your finger over the bead every time you repeat your mantra. Eventually, you'll have moved your fingers over 108 beads, and will know it is time to end your session.

Now is the time to do any scheduling required for your upcoming sessions. Please take a few moments to do this if needed. Stay with the 10-minute session time you did last week (remember to give yourself a few minutes on either side).

For the next seven days, we'll be working with the mantra "Om." This is a great mantra to work with because it's simple, pleasant to say, and highly effective. For each session this week, try to use this technique as described below and notice how well it works for you. Pay attention to how the inclusion of sound energy affects the quality of your meditation.

Following is a step-by-step guide to the method you'll be using this week. You may wish to print out this lesson and carry it with you into your sittings.

OM MEDITATION

Before you begin:

1. Make sure you have on attire that is loose and does not restrict you or makes you uncomfortable.

2. Make sure to ensure minimum distractions by turning off alarms, ringers, televisions, etc.…

3. Prepare your meditation area as needed to your satisfaction. Candles, bells anything that sets the intentions of your practice.

4. Session Time: 10 minutes

Ideally, I would like you to find a place where you can make your chant aloud. If you are unable to do so there are still benefits in repeating it in a soft whisper or in your head. Take a few seconds and loosen your muscles in your jaw and throat.

When you are ready:

1. Take your position and begin to relax. For this particular exercise, it's especially important to make sure your back is straight so you're your lungs have room to fully expand as you speak your mantra. Place your hands on your knees or thighs and open them toward the ceiling, palms heavenward. Take a giant deep breath and let it out. Acknowledge that it is time for your meditation to begin.

2. Now sit and begin to breathe more deeply, drawing the air in slowly and exhaling it at a comfortable rate. Make sure your inhale is coming from your stomach and not your chest. Repeat this a few times.

3. Start repeating your mantra. The word you're saying is Om, pronounced a-u-m. Realistically, it will be strange hearing

your voice used in this manner. If your mind wanders, that's perfectly okay. As soon as you realize your mind has led you somewhere else, release it, breathe deeply, and return to your mantra. Do this every time your awareness wanders and chant for as long as you possibly can.

4. At the end of your session, take a couple of minutes to ground yourself. The act of grounding yourself is just returning to your present moment and once again be conscious of the environment. I want you to focus on the floor underneath you, the bed or mattress, the couch. Think of how it feels on your body. Think of the sensation it gives your hips, back arms etc.…think about the room you are in, wiggle your toes, and return to the present moment.

5. Take a moment and journal how you feel. Write your first experience down, what distractions did your experience? How many times were you able to catch your mind drifting during your session? What thoughts keep coming to you? What are those images that come to mind? I want to talk about these sessions with you at the end of the week so make

sure you join our FB group. Post this week's results in the FB

group

"Peace...inner peace is when your what you display to the world is in perfect alignment with what is inside your heart!"

-Demetrius Irick

]

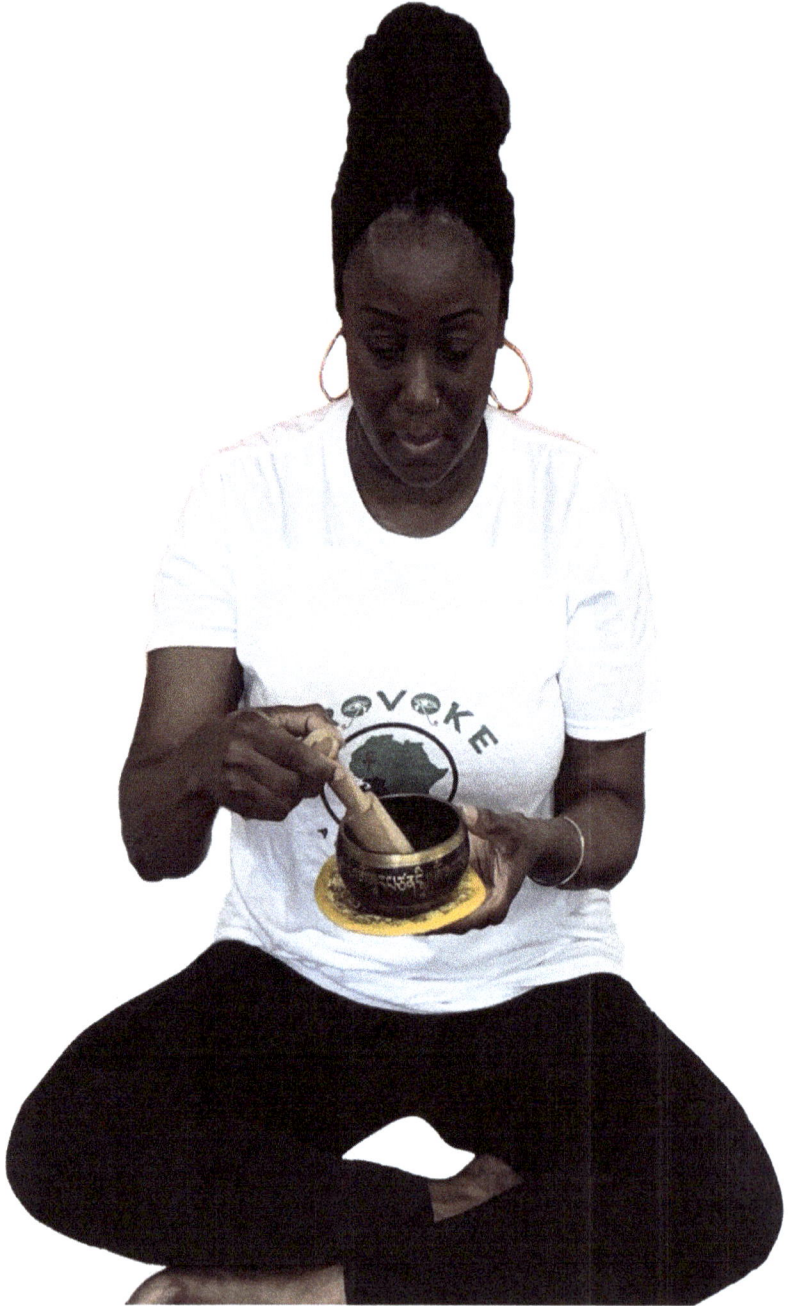

Sound Meditation

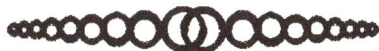

Beginner Meditation

Week 6

EXPLORING MEDITATION THROUGH SOUND (LISTENING)

We will use the sense of sound this week for your practice. When using sound meditation we are using our ears to translate the vibration to our brain. Have you ever listen to a song and you felt it? That's an example of what we will be doing this week.

We will be paying close attention to what we receive from the energy we encounter from vibrations. The sense of hearing is powerful think about the animals that use this sense with such pinpoint accuracy. When we use our sense of hearing with determination, purpose, and intention it becomes extremely effective in its ability to guide us and focus the mind.

Demetrius Irick

Think about this when we were formed in the belly of our mother one of the first senses that was developed was our sense of sound, the observation of our mother's heartbeat and it's rhythmic beat guided us back/forth into consciousness. The steady consistent beat was our guide in complete darkness and we became content with its place in our life. We connected to the vibration, getting agitated when the mother was agitated, getting a boost of energy when mom was exerting herself. Our life as we knew it was centered on a strong, steady heartbeat.

Many of the ancient cultures have long since understood the benefit of using sound in its progress to focus the mind. The Ancient civilizations like Native American, African, and Chinese use sound as key avenues for focusing of the mind to higher levels of consciousness. Archaeologists have uncovered musical instruments like flutes carved of bone that date back to the prehistoric era. This connection to music has a primal connection with us as humans and is another example of how music or sound calms our mind.

The benefits of listening to music include the management of stress on the mind and body. When you add meditation and music you get the most out of a deeper concentration and focus. Many forms of music can be used to assist in meditation. The choices of waterfalls, nature, birds chirping anything that will give your mind comfort. I suggest staying away from songs that trigger painful memories.

Earlier, we spoke of the importance of establishing consistency in our practice, by meditating in the same place, and same time if possible, lighting a candle or incense to spark a routine. It's a good idea as well when it comes to sounds or music selections during your sessions. When you have become more grounded in your practice adding additional types of music to your practice will generate different thoughts, emotional vibrations, triggers, and feeling so be prepared to do the work that it will present. Always, be prepared to seek clarity in the thoughts and emotions that come up during your sessions because only you can unlock its inner meaning to your life

The purpose of having a practice of music selection is to help you get into a meditative state quickly. The African drumbeat is perhaps the most primal and captivating of all rhythms. Perhaps this is because of its similarity to the sound of a heartbeat; after all, our first introduction to sound was in the womb where the rhythm of our mother's heartbeat eased our transition into form.

In many cultures, the beating of a drum gets the listener's minds quickly into another state or realm. It's used in ceremonies and part of the healing process or rituals for the souls of participants. Even to this day people get into what called a drum circle and use the transformative sound of the drum to meditative states of consciousness.

Studies also show that drum meditation can support the treatment of some diseases and also reduce depression, curb memory loss. Several years ago, the drum was an important component of Buddhist tradition as it is used to gather everyone into a sacred place where the precept of the worship will be relayed to practitioners. The drumbeats bring mindful clarity to all the puzzles of the mind especially when it is accompanied by chanting.

Singing Bowls

The Tibetan singing bowl has been used by practicing Buddhists to help them reach meditative states of meditation. When the user guides the mallet around the surface of the bowl it produces a sound. It has been used to start and end the meditation when a tap of the bowl is given.

When the user pressing the mallet against the bowl in a slow circular manner it produces a beautiful sound that can be controlled by the speed of the movement of the mallet. I've personally found the singing bowls to quickly whipped me

Demetrius Irick

off into meditative states and recommend them in your practice.

The sound is usually cleared, bright, and enchanting. Always strike the bowl before you begin the circular motion at the outside belly of the bowl.
Singing bowls are an extremely effective way to enlist the help of our senses in calming our mind.

This week, your meditation tool will be music. Some ideas might be traditional meditation music such as the ragas, drumming, and singing bowls described above, in addition to chanting…YouTube has some great meditative music as well.

You might want to print out this lesson to bring into your session.

MUSIC MEDITATION

Before you begin:

1. Make sure you have on attire that is loose and does not restrict you or makes you uncomfortable.

2. Make sure to ensure minimum distractions by turning off alarms, ringers, televisions, etc....

3. Prepare your meditation area as needed to your satisfaction. Candles, bells anything that sets the intentions of your practice.

4. Session Time: 10 minutes

5. Set up your music of choice

When you are ready:_

1. Press play on the music.

2. Take your position and begin to relax. Place your hand on your knees or thighs and open them up towards the ceiling, palms heavenward (ready to receive the blessings of the universe). Take a giant deep breath and let it out. Acknowledge that this is now your meditation time.

3. Now sit and begin to breathe more deeply, drawing the air in slowly and exhaling it at a comfortable rate. Make sure your inhale is coming from your stomach and not your chest. Repeat this a few times.

4. Now, close your eyes and feel the vibration of the music as it reaches your outer skin. Listen to the music with your ears, with every fiber of your body as it travels through your being. Pay close attention to the energy as it penetrates your body and causes sensations throughout your physical body. Try to focus on the rhythm of the song that is playing.

 If your mind wanders, just keep bringing yourself back to the music. Use the Power of 5 breathing technique to guide you back to the sounds and to regain focus. Breathe deeply, release your thoughts, and listen. Do this every time your awareness leaves the music and the present moment.

5. At the end of your session, take a couple of minutes to ground yourself. The act of grounding yourself is just returning to your present moment and once again be conscious of the environment. I want you to feel the floor underneath you, the bed or mattress, the couch. Think of how it feels on your body. Think of the sensation it gives your hips,

back arms etc....think about the room you are in, wiggle your toes, and return to the present moment.

6. Take a moment and journal how you feel. Write your first experience down, what distractions did your experience? How many times were you able to catch your mind drifting during your session? What thoughts keep coming to you? What are those images that come to mind? I want to talk about these sessions with you at the end of the week so make sure you join our FB group. Post this week's results in the FB group

*"**Keep it Real!** is a term people of color say often yet the realest thing you can do is keep it real with yourself. Setting boundaries and keeping commitments, you set for yourself creates the discipline needed to honor your word to others. I will keep it real with myself so I can keep it **REAL** to others!"*

-Demetrius Irick

Demetrius Irick

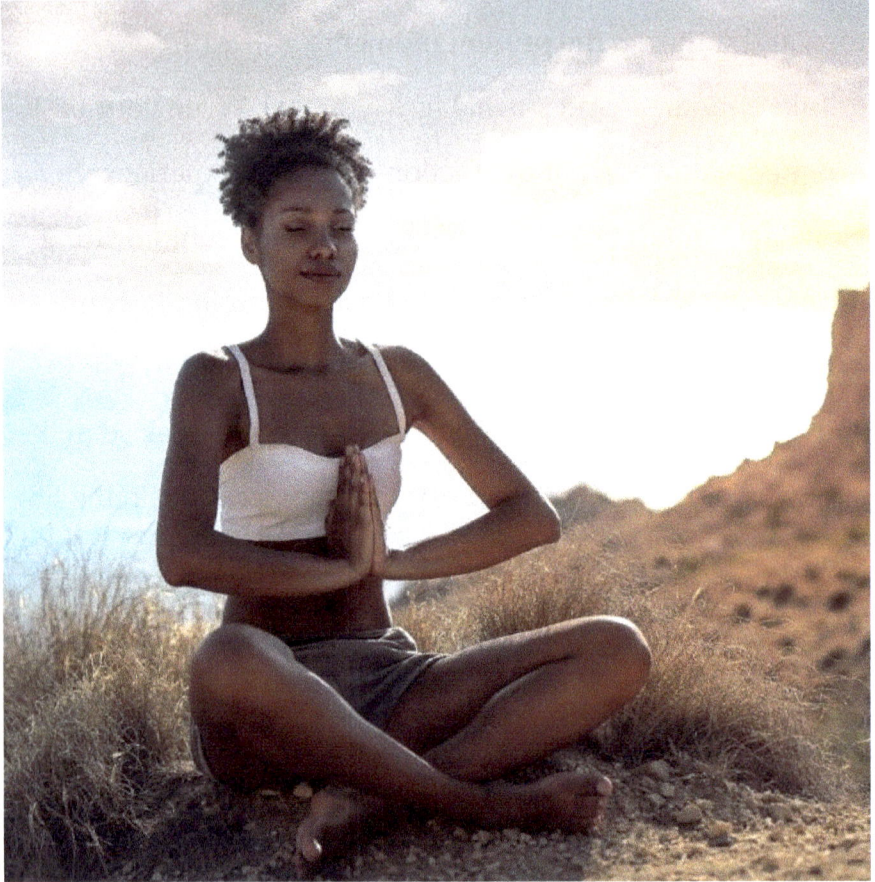

" *Sometimes we get complacent in our lives…things are on autopilot and seem that everything is perfect. I've found that to be the point in my life when there was no growth.*"

-*Demetrius Irick*

Meditation Through Movement

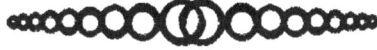

Beginner Meditation

Week 7

This week we're going to be exploring a different kind of meditation. All this week I want you to find someplace that you can walk comfortably and safely or look into some yoga movements. This exercise will allow all your lessons from our previous weeks to come together. You will use a combination of all of your senses during this walking or yoga meditation.

MEDITATION THROUGH MOVEMENT

So far, we've worked with several different techniques to help us cultivate mental discipline. We've explored methods that isolate different senses and ones that appeal to multiple senses at once. This week we'll be exploring meditation through physical movement, which, because our whole bodies are involved, necessitates an awareness of our inner experience as well as the outer terrain. If effective, you may begin to experience the world inside and around you with absolute presence. This week you will be introduced to three new ways of using your skills.

1.) Walking Meditations

Walking meditations tend to be perfect for individuals who find it difficult to sit for long periods. The process of walking or yoga involves physical, mental, and emotional energy to add to your arsenal of sources for inner peace. I've found that walking outside especially around nature seems to be the most profound experience for me but ultimately you must find what works best for you. My clients have various experience levels and live in a multitude of areas therefore only you can determine the best travel location that is safe. Whether walking in a park, forest, beach, or a busy sidewalk in a major city it works the same. I found myself walking in my house doing several laps when the weather wasn't great for outside adventure. I found the true test was being present with every step noticing your breath, environment, sounds, and smells as you move throughout your walk.

Tips:

When a person is taking a meditative walk on the road; he or she must be careful and pay close attention to road warnings to avoid accidents. In essence, wherever you've decided to take the walk, you must make sure it is safe enough to protect yourself during your walk. When taking a walk, you should consider the following points: Secure a location that will allow you to take a walk back and forth safely and make sure the environment is peaceful.

Try to focus your attention on both internal and external sensations that flash through the mind while the breath is coming in and out of you. At this moment you should be careful enough to interpret the images that come to mind notating them and filing them mentally until you can place them in your journal.

When you discover that your mind wanders keep calm, it is normal for such to occur, what you'll do is to refocus on those positive sensations going through your body. Refocus on the breath, the feelings in your legs, the wind on your skin, and the air as it flows off your face. You can do the Power of 5 breathing technique to get you back into alignment and focused. Find a way to incorporate this process of walking to your life. You will be amazed at how this little exercise will help you towards inner peace.

Remember your attention should be focused on being, rather than on arriving, be in the moment. You become mindful of your breathing and hold your eyes with a soft gaze. From the first step to the last, each foot is placed with intent. When you are walking find a natural rhythm that corresponds with your breathing pattern.

2.) Mudras

Mudras originated within Kemetic traditions and are gestures and attitudes expressed through hand positions. Although, associated with Indian and Buddhist traditions sculptures on the walls of the pyramid confirm that it's origin begun in Kemet and migrated out of Egypt to other areas.

The word "mudra" means to seal or symbol. There are hundreds of mudra positions. All of them are seen as keys to open up higher states of awareness. When a mudra is performed, your physical, emotional, mental, and spiritual system can open up to reaching a new higher meditative state.

As you begin meditating with these concepts, focus on performing physical tasks like mudras can help calm and steady your mind.

When performing a Mudra the fingers are placed in certain positions, pressing on points in the hand that affect different parts of the body and psyche. Each mudra can be thought of as an expression of an enlightened mental or emotional state that you might seek to embody.

Demetrius Irick

The Sanskrit term is a seal of ideas and codes connecting bodily signs with the brain. The hands can be seen as part of the sensory reception from the outside world that connects the movement of the hands with the brain. As such it can be interpreted that the shapes or sign that the hands form is the workings of our mind and a great measurement of the kind of energy flow that is on. When you use the hands outward, it is believed that you're drawing yourself inward as well. The mudras techniques have a way of contributing to the bodily health and empower the level of human thinking.

3.) Martial Arts & Yoga

Tai Chi & Yoga are two other forms of movement meditations. These forms of meditation use movement exercise to focus and quiet the mind. It's entirely too many forms of martial arts & yoga to discuss all of them but require the practitioners to such within. Both martial arts and yoga brings awareness to the breath, energy and it's flow through the body.

In both practices the understanding that the core energy center is in the navel area and is the essence of our being.

Practicing martial arts and yoga require a degree of self-control, clearing the mind of distractions, negative thoughts that hinder the progress of the participant. Yoga practices are designed to train the mind to maintain focus, minimizes random thoughts, and reveals deep emotions that lie beneath the surface.

Continuing Your Meditation Practice

We've covered a lot of ground this week. Hopefully, you're not feeling overwhelmed but are instead excited about the many options available to you. We talked at the beginning of the book about how establishing a practice of meditating will help you become a healthier stronger individual. All of these different techniques that we've been covering are simply possibilities for you to learn about and consider in your ongoing growth and development. The more you know, the better able you are to customize your practice and create the best routine possible.

As you plan your meditations for the week, see if you can increase your time. You're going to choose one of the above moving meditations to work with throughout the seven days. I suggest a basic walking meditation to start being mindful of everything through the session. Next, try one of the other practices a yoga pose or Mudra.

1. Make sure you have on attire that is loose and does not restrict you or makes you uncomfortable.

2. Make sure to ensure minimum distractions by turning off alarms, ringers, televisions, etc.…

3. Prepare your meditation area as needed to your satisfaction. Candles, bells anything that sets the intentions of your practice.

4. Session Time: 15 minutes

When you are ready:

1. Take your position and begin to relax if you are doing a Mudra. Place your hand on your knees or thighs and open them up towards the ceiling, palms heavenward (ready to receive the blessings of the universe). Take a giant deep

breath and let it out. Acknowledge that this is now your meditation time.

2. Now sit and begin to breathe more deeply, drawing the air in slowly and exhaling it at a comfortable rate. Make sure your inhale is coming from your stomach and not your chest. Repeat this a few times.

3. Throughout the session, pay attention to your breathing. Feel the relationship between the rate of your breath and the rhythmic movement of your muscles as you walk. If your mind wanders, just keep bringing yourself back to your breath and the movement of your body. If you're someplace in nature, you can also experiment with tuning into natural sounds such as birds singing or wind rustling through the leaves. If you are practicing yoga or martial arts technique close attention should be taken account of the breathing of each movement.

4. If you are doing a walking meditation please consider the safety precaution discuss at the beginning of this week. When you are through, take the time to ground yourself.

5. At the end of your session, take a couple of minutes to ground yourself. The act of grounding yourself is just returning to your present moment and once again be conscious of the environment. I want you to focus on the floor underneath you, the bed or mattress, the couch. Think of how it feels on your body. Think of the sensation it gives your hips, back arms etc.…think about the room you are in, wiggle your toes, and return to the present moment.

6. Take a moment and journal how you feel. Write your first experience down, what distractions did your experience? How many times were you able to catch your mind drifting during your session? What thoughts keep coming to you? What are those images that come to mind? I want to talk about these sessions with you at the end of the week so make sure you join our FB group. Post this week's results in the FB group.

"Your spirit is yearning to be at peace...sit still and listen to what the voice inside has to say and you will find the peace you desire."

-Demetrius Irick

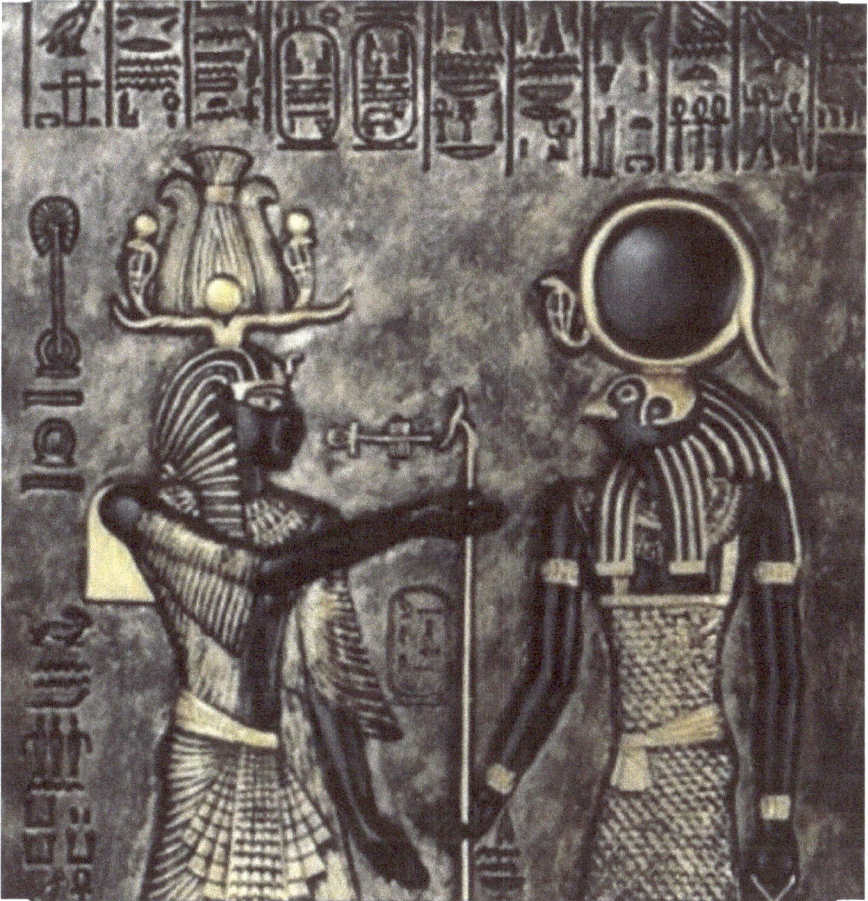

"It's those days that you want to skip your practice that will make the most out of your practice!"

-Demetrius Irick

Demetrius Irick

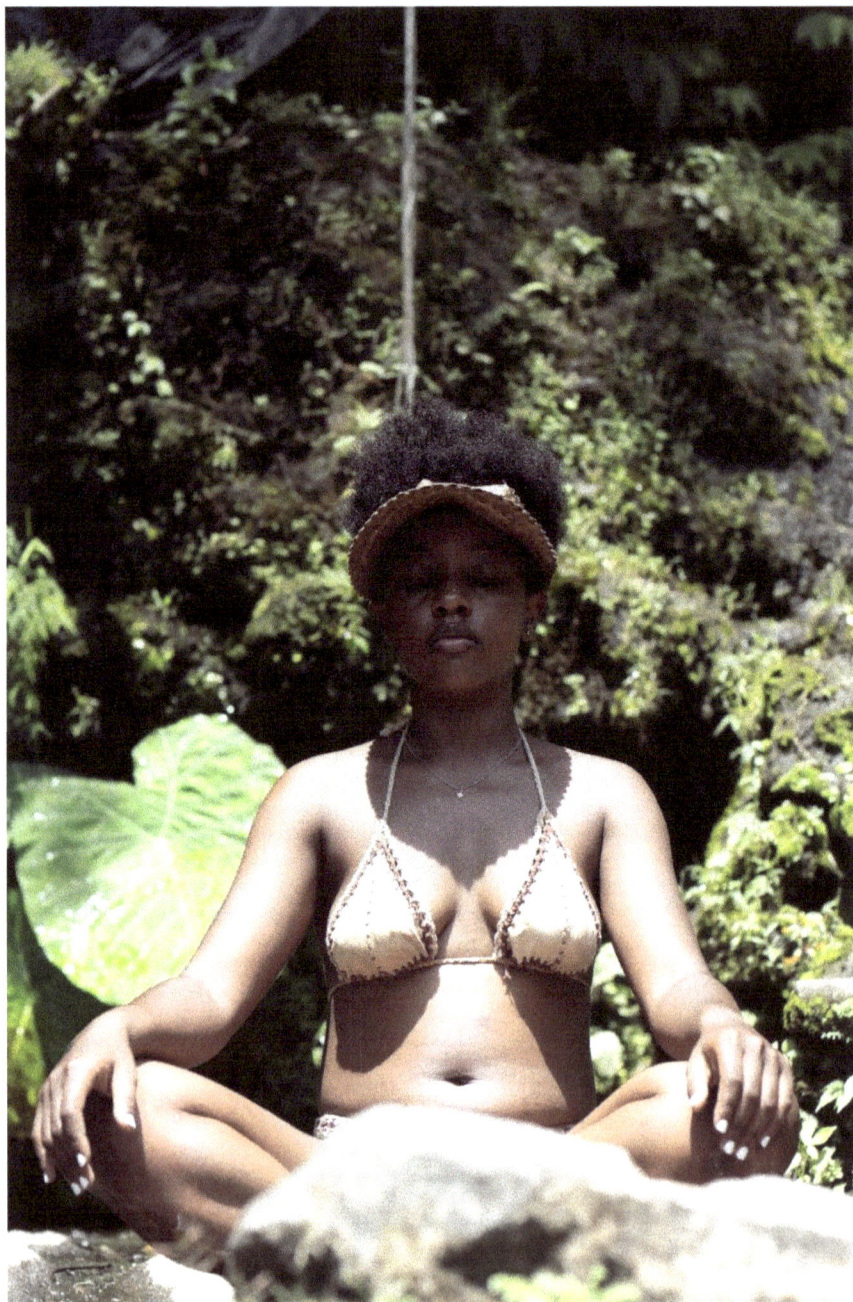

Meditation Through Nature

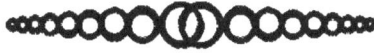

Beginner Meditation

Week 8

This is our final lesson. We've been exploring meditation for seven weeks now and you've probably developed a pretty good sense of what works for you. You know how your monkey mind responds to the different techniques and have hopefully determined at least one method that helps tame it. Think back to when you first started this journey. It is probably quite easier for you to meditate now than it was when you began. Take a second and just tell yourself...thank you! Thank your higher self for sticking with the process and not given up on an activity that will enhance your life.

 Do you notice that you look forward to your sessions? Have you found a difference in your day when you skip a session? Have you noticed your emotional highs and lows throughout the week? Maybe you find it easier to shift into a meditative zone than you did before. Also, consider how your life may feel different outside of the meditation sessions themselves. Are you more confident in what you want? Are you able to resolve conflicts and disagreements without it ruining your whole day? Are you able to deal with stressful situations just a little bit better today? Yeah! It's working...congrats!

I want you to take a minute and just be grateful for your progress thus far. Pat yourself on the back for the progress you've made. Give yourself a few minutes to appreciate how far you've come.

Now, that you have come this far you will notice that you have come to have a greater appreciation for nature. It's something remarkable that when we find that we are becoming more balance in our life we understand how nature gives us peace spiritually. We tend to have a newfound respect for the creatures of the wild, their freedoms, and how the universe provides everything they need to survive. We tend to get a better understanding of how unbalanced our lives have been until meditation brought that awareness back into our lives.

I feel such a connection when I am with nature whether it's sitting in my backyard and listening to the birds or watching the squirrels run from tree to tree. The feeling that nature provides gives my soul an inner peace. I've found personally that connecting with nature to be the ultimate form of meditation, the purest form of the state of being, and pure awareness. This week we're going to incorporate what we've learned over the recent weeks and discuss the role that nature can play to enhance our meditation practices. The week ahead can be thought of as a journey to a place of deep familiarity. Even if we've lived in the city our whole life, there will always be a part of us that feels greater peace by connecting with the beauty of nature.

In modern times we think ourselves as separate from nature, and yet it simply isn't possible. Every cell of our body is filled with water. The trees have purified every breath we take for

Demetrius Irick

us. Every piece of food we eat has, in some way, come from the earth. Our separation from nature is only an illusion, a mental construct much like many of our other thoughts about whom we are and what we're here on earth to accomplish. Meditation has helped us to discover these connections.

The human soul has direct connections with every living being on this planet to include: plants, animals, and mother earth herself. When you think about the human being in general on a grand scale the human being had a greater connection to the land. We lived off the land-only using what we needed, giving thanks to the land that provided everything to sustain life. In recent centuries our level of respect for nature has decreased and we are abusing our connection with mother earth. When we find ourselves in nature it's a deep spiritual yearning that has been fulfilled. There is a feeling of being home to our soul because we are interconnected.

The connection to the natural world reminds us to be in the now...appreciating the moment. I am a dog lover and every dog I've ever had has always greeted me with such love and joy that I wish humans could replicate. No matter what might have happened prior to, the love that is displayed is genuine. Any pet owner to relate to this love animals give their owners the same love is felt when we are in nature. Some of us are naturally drawn to animals simply because of the way that being near them makes us feel balanced. Qi Gong, a Taoist meditative practice actually uses animal movements to achieve harmony in their bodies. Some of the postures are the crane, bear, and goose to name a few...these animals in their natural environment possessed a level of awareness which led to them studying their lives.

When we spend quality time in nature our spirits are re-awakened, refreshed, and screams more, more. Something as simple as walking barefooted has been proven to reduce depression and anxiety...crazy right? The healing powers of our connection with nature are still being explored and examined for all its rewards. Think of how peaceful you get walking on a beach, on a beautiful sunny day, and the feeling of serenity it provides. Meditation provides the same feeling of peace.

Shamanic Gaze

Some shamanic traditions practice a walking meditation similar to the ones we recently learned about. This meditation, however, is always done in nature. The meditator softens their focused awareness by expanding vision to include awareness of the peripheral landscape. This assists in creating a more expansive, inclusive mind.

Listening

Sometimes a meditation with nature can be as simple as sitting with a stone, a leaf, or other objects from nature in front of you and listening with your inner ear, your heart, and soul. The practice involves allowing the object to speak in its stillness and silence, connecting you with the depth of the messages and wisdom of the soul. This wisdom need not come in the form of words; rather, it can be a calm, harmonious presence...just be. This technique is wonderful for tree lovers too. You can sit next to the same tree every day and build a relationship over time that provides a remarkable depth of meditative awareness and natural communion.

Garden Meditation

Have you ever thought about starting a garden? The smell of spearmint, lemon balm, lavender, and rosemary can provide unique smells that send you on a meditative state. The joy of cultivating and being with the soil, plants, water, sun forms a bond that only mother nature can deliver. Make your meditation garden a relaxing space to envision, listen, observe, and receive messages from Source.

NATURE MEDITATION

After this week you'll be on your own to continue your regular chosen practice of meditation. Hopefully, you'll have found a method that suits you well, and hopefully, you'll be willing to grow and evolve it as time goes on.

Demetrius Irick

For me, some of my best meditations occur outside in nature. I feel so supported by plants, animals, mountains, and oceans. I watch for signals, what bug lands on me, what crosses my pass. I can watch ants, squirrels, and birds for hours. I pay close attention to the closeness I feel to them and they to me. I listen to the leaves and the music they play as the wind blows shuffling them. I welcome all messages that the universe is offering and claim the wisdom of the ages. For this final week, you'll be exploring an open-eyed meditation in nature. Even if your climate makes this idea somewhat unappealing, think of ways you could make it more enjoyable. This can be one of your most rewarding meditations experienced yet, so give it a try.

You might want to print out this lesson to bring into your session.

Before you begin:

1. Put on some comfortable, weather-appropriate clothing that will not bind while you are sitting.

2. Leave your cell phone behind if you can. If you must have it with you, turn it off for your meditation.

3. Select the location for your meditation. It should be somewhere that is comfortable to sit or stand-in for a period of time. This means that you'll be shaded from the hot sun or protected from a chilling wind.

4. Determine what your focal point will be. Choose an item or a scene that feels calming for you. Avoid selecting an animal such as a bird or a squirrel as your focal point, since the animal may eventually leave the scene.

When you are ready:

1. Get in a place where you feel comfortable. Locate your item of focus and whether sitting or standing be cognizant of your environment. If you standing it's important to ensure your feet are at least shoulder-width apart and give your knees a slight bend to prevent locking your legs.

2. Now begin to relax. If sitting, place your hands on your knees or thighs and open them toward the ceiling, palms heavenward. If standing, simply relax your arms by your sides. Take a giant deep breath and let it out. Acknowledge that it is time for your meditation to begin.

3. Now with your eyes two-thirds of the way open, your gaze soft and held naturally on the item or scene you've chosen simply remains still and breath. For the entire length of your session, just breathe and focus on your item. Use the Power of 5 breathing technique. Feel free to blink softly and naturally. Make no judgment on what happens. Your mind may wander and that's perfectly okay. As soon as you realize your mind has led you somewhere else, release it, and breathe deeply. Do this every time your awareness leaves the present moment.

4. At the end of your session, take a couple of minutes to ground yourself. The act of grounding yourself is just returning to your present moment and once again be conscious of the environment. The ground underneath you, the three, bench or ground. Think of how it feels on your body. Think of the sensation it gives your hips, back arms

etc....think about the smells around you and comes back to your current reality.

5. Take a moment and journal how you feel. Write your first experience down, what distractions did your experience? How many times were you able to catch your mind drifting during your session? What thoughts keep coming to you? What are those images that come to mind? I want to talk about these sessions with you at the end of the week so make sure you join our FB group. Post this week's results in the FB group

Final Thoughts

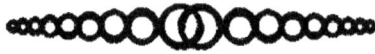

After you've finished this week's meditation practice in nature, continue meditating with the practice that fits your lifestyle the best.

The longer you meditate, the more we begin to see opportunities for life itself to become a living meditation. If you find yourself in a difficult situation in life, remember that you can always draw upon the feeling you have while meditating and you'll instantly feel more grounded and centered. Meditation is yet another tool in your toolbox of life to use whenever you need it.

I hope that you have Peace, Blessings and Light!

Life

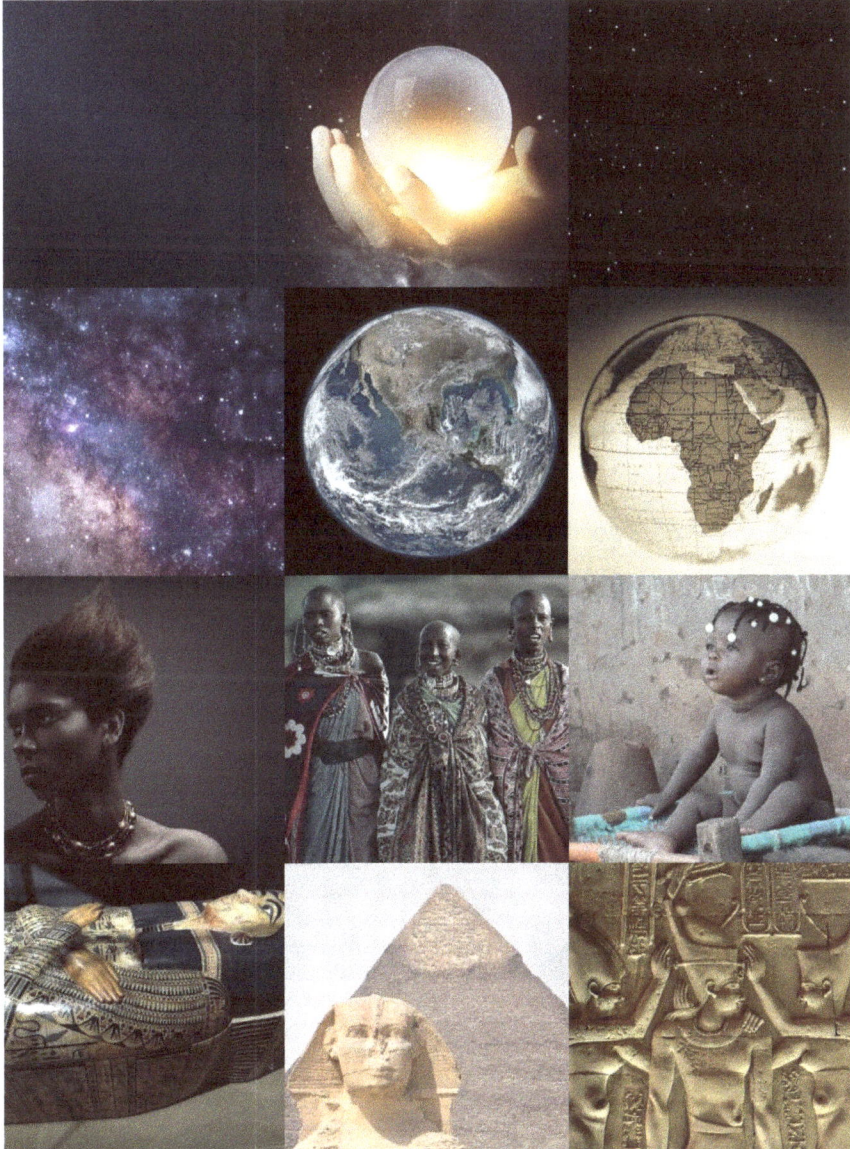

Demetrius Irick

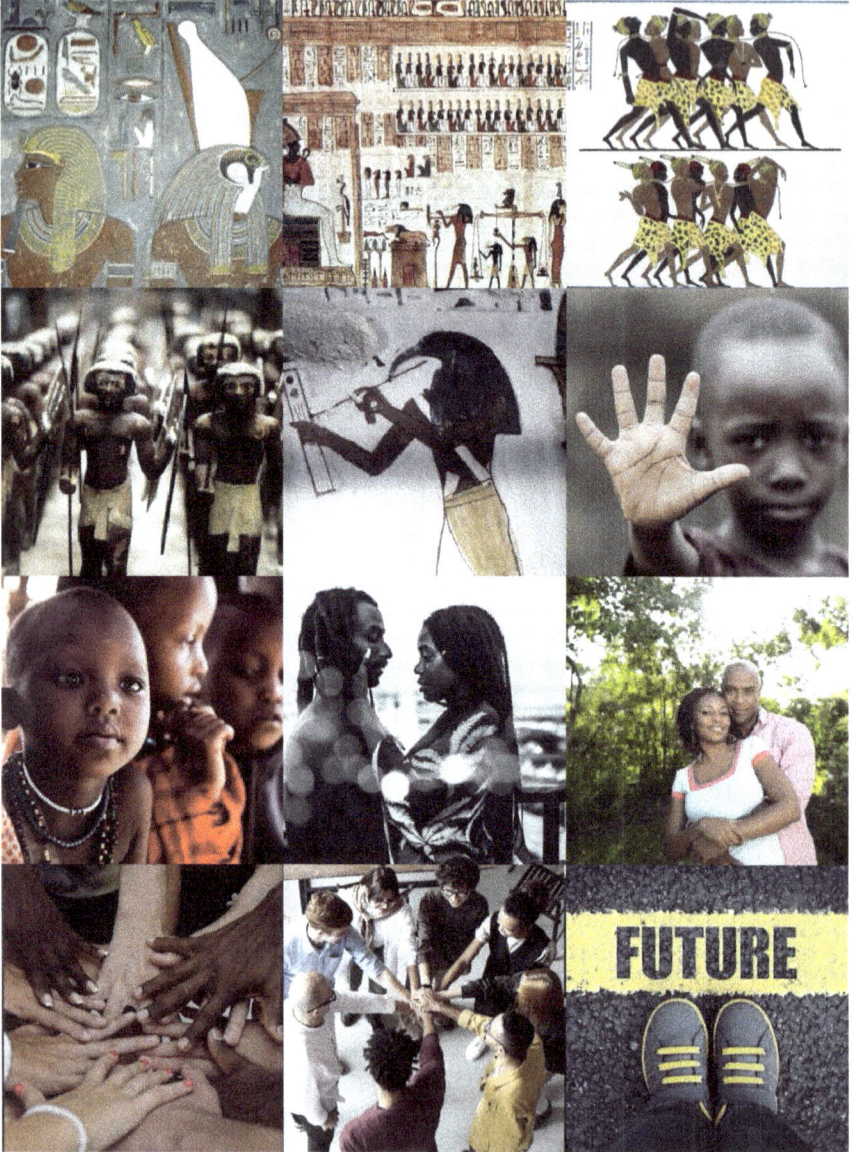

Bonus Meditations

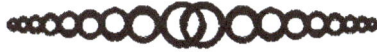

Belly Full

Session: 5-10 minutes

1. Lay flat on your back on the floor

2. Close your eyes or soften your gaze on an item

3. Pay attention to your breath. Take five deep breaths, only focus on the inhale and exhale & it's natural rhythm.

4. As you observe this process...start feeling where in your body do your feel physical sensations, your nose, rib cage, belly, knees, etc.

5. Place your hands on your belly and the other hand on your chest.

6. Bring your awareness to the points where your hands have pressure on your chest and stomach. Scan the area of those points of your body.

7. Bring your awareness back to your stomach, deep inhale, and exhale. Move your hands back along your side.

8. Repeat to yourself aloud…I AM Grateful…I AM Blessed…five times.

9. Ground yourself…returning to your day.

Mindful Eating

Session: 5-10 minutes

1. Select the item you will eat…preferably a piece of fruit for the demonstration.

2. Make sure you sit to a table is possible that is clear of anything except the item of choice.

3. Declare to the universe you will eat this fruit mindfully enjoying every fiber of the item and the sensations it has on my body.

4. Observe the item, take in all of it's physical attributes before touching it. Look at the colors, is the surface smooth, lumpy, ridget?

5. Pickup the item and inhale deeply, three times try observing the smell of the fruit. Does it have a smell? Is it sweet? What are you able to pickup using your sense of smell?

6. Bring the fruit directly touching your nose now and repeat #5. Observe the texture of the fruit as it touches your skin, as you inhale what sensations runs through your body…what thoughts come to your mind? What emotions are generated…are you getting excited? Hungry? Be patient

7. Now, is the time to taste it…Open you eyes and take a nice size bite, closing your eyes after. Hmmm, taste it as it swirls around your mouth, How, does it feel on your tongue? What do you taste? What enters your mind after the prolonged process, desire to eat it?

8. Now, as you swallow, follow it down the body, noticing it as it travels throughout your body. Notice the points it travels from your mouth, throat and everywhere in between.

9. Continue eating your fruit in this manner until you are finished. After you have completed this exercise think about the entire process and how was it different from you eating normally?

Sources

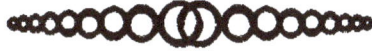

Harvard Business Review:

https://hbr.org/2015/01/mindfulness-can-literally-change-your-brain

(Accessed 5/19/20)

National Institution of Health:

Mindfulness practice leads to increases in regional brain gray matter density

https://www.ncbi.nlm.nih.gov/pmc/articles/PMC3004979/

(Accessed 5/19/20)

National Library of Medicine:

Mindfulness Based Intervention in Parkinson's Disease Leads to Structural Brain Changes on MRI

https://pubmed.ncbi.nlm.nih.gov/24184066/

(Accessed 5/19/20)

National Library of medicine:

Demetrius Irick

Mindfulness Practice Leads to Increases in Regional Brain

Gray Matter Density

https://pubmed.ncbi.nlm.nih.gov/21071182/

(Accessed 5/19/2020)

Journal of Alternative and Complementary Medicine:

Therapeutic Potential of a Drum and Dance Ceremony based

on the African Ngoma Tradition

https://www.ncbi.nlm.nih.gov/pmc/articles/PMC4523073/
(Accessed 8/9/2020)

Schneider, Dr. Robert. "Does Meditation Have Benefits for
Mind and Body? " Medical New Today. February 26, 2014.
https://www.medicalnewstoday.com/articles/272833
(Accessed 8/11/2020)

Schulte, Brigid. "Harvard Neuroscientist: Meditation Not Only
Reduces Stress, Here's How It Changes Your Brain."
Washington Post. May 26, 2015.
https://www.washingtonpost.com/news/inspired-
life/wp/2015/05/26/harvard-neuroscientist-meditation-not-only-
reduces-stress-it-literally-changes-your-
brain/?utm_term=.dd361811a8e5.
(Accessed 8/11/2020)

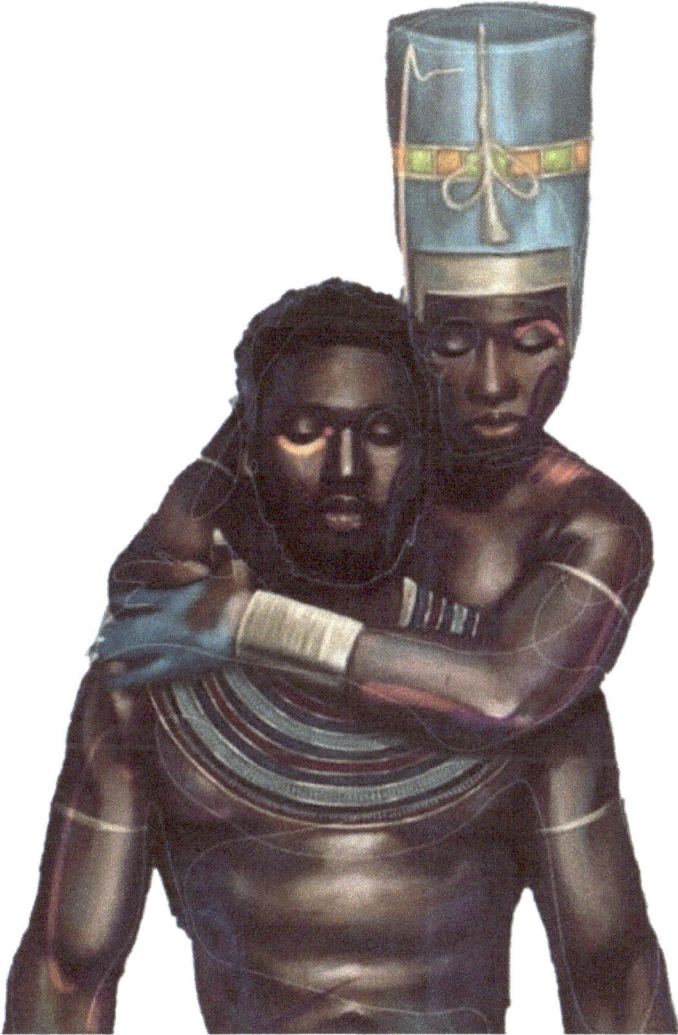

Demetrius Irick

Facebook Group:

https://www.facebook.com/akiliflow

Website:

www.akiliflow.com

Apps:

Insight timer

Headspace

Brightmind

YouTube:

www.youtube.com/akiliflow

www.youtube.com/lovemeditation

Books

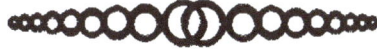

Stay Woke

-Justin, Michael Williams

Egyptian Yoga, Postures of the Gods and Goddesses

-Muata Ashby

Meditation: The Ancient Egyptian Path to Enlightenment

-Muata Ashby

Glorious Light Meditation

-Muata Ashby

Meditation for relaxation

-Adam o Neil

The Art of Living

-Thich Nhat Hann

21 Days of Guided Meditation

-Jess Ray

10% Happier

-Dan Harris

Power of Habit

-Charles Duhigg

Daily Self-Discipline

-Martin Meadows

About the Author

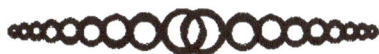

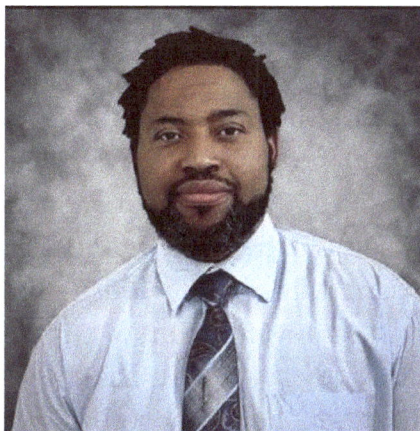

If you want to have a solid meditation practice you have to do the work and practice. In this book, your coach Demetrius Irick presents informative guidance about different techniques, the history, and instructions on exploring meditation for beginners. The journey is explored with a different technique for each week as you are given clear, step-by-step instructions to building their practice. The meditative practices presented in this book will give you peace, serenity, better sleep, and reduce stress or anxiety that plague most humans in our current fast-paced world. Meditation is great for leaders, mothers, executives, and anyone in between. This book will offer the reader down to earth information that will benefit newcomers and experienced meditators alike. If you are ready to be at peace with your thoughts, engage in a quick meditation so you can enjoy the immediate effects of this practice.

Demetrius Irick

Demetrius Irick is a meditation coach, a social activist, Co-Founder of AkiliFlow, a Certified Professional & Executive Coaching Organization & Provoke Press, an independent self-publishing company designed to help first-time authors get their books published. Demetrius at his core believes his destiny is tied to helping individuals, couples, and organizations to reach their optimal performance using the Art of Meditation and Kemetic Yoga™□ as foundational principles and tools. Demetrius, a serial entrepreneur and best selling author of "I'm Finally a Man, A husband's Journey to Manhood, has dedicated his life to the development of people and their God-given talents. Equipped with a pure passion to serve others his mission is to help others begin the journey of becoming the best version of themselves reaching their spiritual, physical and life goals.

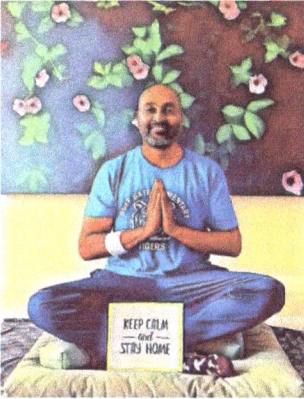

Follow Mr. Stevey on Instagram

Mr. Stevey promotes mindfulness for children, teens and adults. Follow his page for motivation and tips to enhance your life and your children.

IG:@mr_stevey_meditates

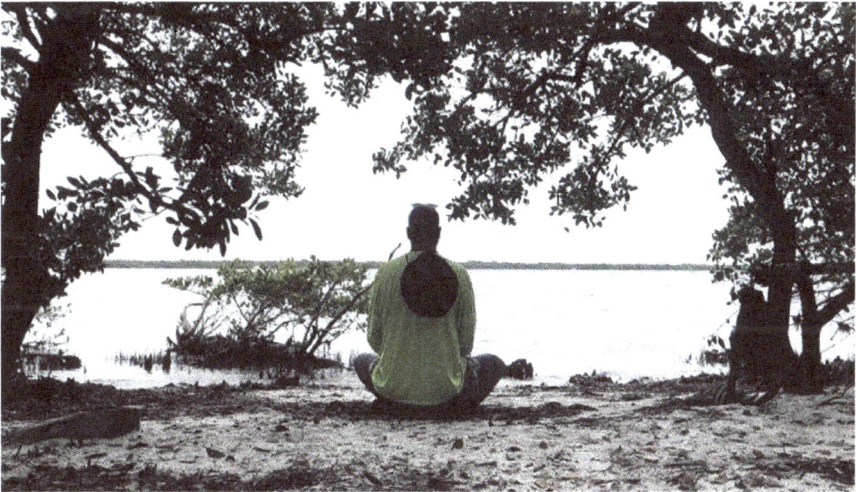

" Life with all of its diversity, complexities and laughter is really as simple as your next breath. Take the time to appreciate your breath and your life will be at PEACE!"

-Demetrius Irick

www.ingramcontent.com/pod-product-compliance
Lightning Source LLC
Chambersburg PA
CBHW071541040426
42452CB00008B/1080